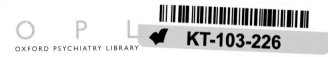

OXFORD PSYCHIATRY LIBRARY

KT-103-226

Panic Disorder and Agoraphobia

O P L

OXFORD PSYCHIATRY LIBRARY

Panic Disorder and Agoraphobia

Prof. Dr. Borwin Bandelow

Department of Psychiatry and Psychotherapy, University of Göttingen
Göttingen, Germany

Prof. Dr. Dr. Katharina Domschke

Department of Psychiatry, Psychosomatics and Psychotherapy,
University of Würzburg, Würzburg, Germany

Prof. David S. Baldwin

Clinical and Experimental Sciences (CNS and Psychiatry),
Faculty of Medicine, University of Southampton
Southampton, UK

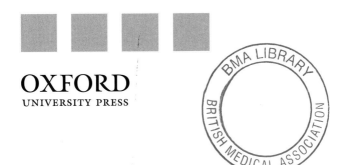

OXFORD
UNIVERSITY PRESS

OXFORD
UNIVERSITY PRESS

Great Clarendon Street, Oxford, OX2 6DP,
United Kingdom

Oxford University Press is a department of the University of Oxford.
It furthers the University's objective of excellence in research, scholarship,
and education by publishing worldwide. Oxford is a registered trade mark of
Oxford University Press in the UK and in certain other countries

First Edition published in 2014

Impression: 1

Published in the United States of America by Oxford University Press
198 Madison Avenue, New York, NY 10016, United States of America

British Library Cataloguing in Publication Data
Data available

Library of Congress Control Number: 2013938538

ISBN 978–0–19–956229–9

Printed in Great Britain
by Ashford Colour Press Ltd, Gosport, Hampshire

Contents

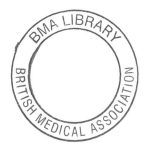

Preface

Fear must be separated into 'realistic' and 'unrealistic' fear. Realistic fear is a normal reaction to a threatening situation and includes fear of car accidents, illnesses, the death of a close relative, terror, war, financial losses, or unemployment. These fears, however, are not normally the reasons why people seek professional help. Anxiety disorders are characterized by unrealistic or inappropriate fears (e.g. the fear of lifts, shopping malls, telephone calls, or mice) or in the case of generalized anxiety disorder, exaggerated fears of real dangers. In contrast to the fear of real dangers, pathological anxiety is not advantageous in the Darwinian sense.

Individuals with panic disorder suffer from recurrent attacks with intense fear, which may occur 'out of the blue' or in special situations, such as crowded places. It typically causes a substantial impairment of social and occupational function.

Patients with panic disorder are not only seen in psychiatric settings, but are also encountered very frequently in primary care. Recognition and adequate treatment of this condition may improve clinical outcomes and quality of life in these patients.

Borwin Bandelow,
Katharina Domschke,
David Baldwin
February 2013

Symbols and abbreviations

5-HT	5-hydroxytryptamine—serotonin
ACTH	Adrenocorticotropic hormone (corticotropin)
CBT	Cognitive behavioural therapy
CRH	Corticotropin releasing hormone
DBPC	Double-blind placebo-controlled study
DBS	Deep brain stimulation
ECT	Electroconvulsive therapy
GAD	Generalized anxiety disorder
HAMA	Hamilton Anxiety Rating Scale
MAOI	Monoamine oxidase inhibitor
NARI	Noradrenaline (norepinephrine) reuptake inhibitor
NaSSA	Noradrenergic and specific serotonergic antidepressant
OCD	Obsessive—compulsive disorder
PTSD	Post-traumatic stress disorder
RCT	Randomized controlled trial
rTMS	Repetitive transcranial magnetic stimulation
RIMA	Reversible inhibitor of monoamine oxidase A
SAD	Social anxiety disorder (social phobia)
SNRI	Serotonin norepinephrine reuptake-inhibitor
SSRI	Selective serotonin reuptake-inhibitor
TCA	Tricyclic antidepressant

Chapter 1

Diagnosis

Key points

- Panic attacks are defined as sudden anxiety attacks with at least 4 out of 13 somatic (physical) and psychic (psychological) anxiety symptoms
- Panic disorder is diagnosed when recurrent panic attacks occur or when at least one attack is followed by enduring anticipatory anxiety
- Agoraphobia is the fear and avoidance of crowds, narrow rooms, public transport or other situations, which can be characterized as places in which patients fear that in case a panic attack occurs, medical help would be difficult to obtain.

1.1 Diagnostic criteria for panic attacks

Among the anxiety disorders, three major disorders are associated with substantial impairment in quality of life and high health care utilization: namely social anxiety disorder, panic disorder, and generalized anxiety disorder. Although panic disorder is only the second most prevalent of these conditions, it is associated with the highest health care utilization.

The *Diagnostic and Statistical Manual for Mental Disorders*—Fourth Edition Text Revision (DSM-IV-TR) [http://www.psychiatry.org/practice/dsm] defines a 'panic attack' as a discrete period of intense fear and discomfort, with a specific symptomatology, that develops abruptly and reaches a peak in 10 minutes or less.

Bodily anxiety symptoms are accompanied by psychic (or psychological) symptoms, including fear of dying, discomfort and foreboding of impending danger. Out of the list of 13 symptoms listed in the DSM (APA, 2000), 4 are required to fulfil the definition of a panic attack.

Panic disorder is listed in the DSM-IV-TR as occurring with or without agoraphobia. In the new DSM 5 diagnostic criteria for panic disorder and agoraphobia are referenced and are listed as separate disorders, each with its own set of distinct diagnostic criteria.

Some patients focus on cardiovascular symptoms, such as palpitations, irregular heartbeat, chest pain, and pain in the left arm. Others report 'pseudoneurological' symptoms like dizziness, unsteady gait, and fainting; problems which they assume could arise from a stroke or other neurological condition. In some patients, panic disorder presents with severe hyperventilation attacks. These patients suffer from the feeling of choking, and therefore they increase their breathing frequency. As a consequence of an increase in p_{CO_2}, hypocalcaemia may develop, which in turn can lead to tetany with carpopedal spasms (contraction of the muscles in the hands). Some patients report only somatic symptoms, but no signs of anxiety or fear ('panic without panic').

A panic attack lasts around 30 minutes on average, with a wide variation between 10 seconds and 4 hours. The offset is gradual, sometimes leaving the patient in a drained and exhausted state. During a panic attack, blood pressure and heart rate are only slightly increased, or within the normal range.

The frequency and severity of panic attacks vary widely, from one or two attacks per year to six attacks or more per day. Some individuals have frequent limited-symptom attacks, which are conventionally regarded as attacks with three symptoms or less. Nocturnal panic attacks that awaken an individual from sleep may also occur.

A clinical vignette of a patient with panic disorder and agoraphobia is included in Section 1.5.

1.2 **Agoraphobia**

In the early stages of panic disorder, attacks usually occur unexpectedly. Agoraphobia develops later in approximately two thirds of patients, this being the fear of crowds, narrow rooms, public transport or other typical situations (see Box 1.1). The anticipation of panic attacks and the misconception that panic attacks are potentially danger-ous medical conditions can often lead to agoraphobic avoidance of feared situations. These can be characterized as places in which patients fear that should they experi-ence a sudden panic attack, they might need immediate medical treatment, which could be difficult to obtain. Patients with agoraphobia therefore tend to avoid these situations. They do not go to public meetings, such as shopping malls, stadiums, res-taurants, cinemas, parties, or churches. They avoid using trains, underground systems, buses and aeroplanes, fearing that in the case of a panic attack no doctor would be available. Patients might restrict a walk in their city to within only a short distance of their general practitioner, or would rather take their bicycle or car with them in order to be able to get to the their doctor's practice faster. Many patients prefer to be accompanied by their spouse, relatives, or friends when in these situations, so that these individuals could assist them by calling an emergency service. In some cases of severe agoraphobia, patients become completely housebound, only feeling secure at home, because agoraphobia is severe and generalized to most situations.

Less commonly, agoraphobia can also appear without panic attacks. Panic disorder in the absence of agoraphobia is sometimes referred to as uncomplicated panic dis-order. Approximately two thirds of patients with panic disorder develop comorbid agoraphobia.

1.3 **Anticipatory anxiety**

As panic attacks may occur 'out of the blue', some patients come to live in constant fear of recurrent panic attacks. Some patients, though having only infrequent panic attacks, are severely restricted in their quality of life due to this anticipatory anxiety. In patients with agoraphobia, about 30% of the panic attacks still occur spontaneously, when not in feared situations. Thus, although the patients tend to avoid agoraphobic situations, they typically still live in fear of unexpected panic attacks.

Box 1.1 Agoraphobia: typical feared situations

Supermarkets, shopping malls
Public transport: underground, buses, trains, ships, aeroplanes
Crowds, parties or other social gatherings, restaurants
Theatres, cinemas
Auditoriums, stadiums
Classrooms, lecture theatres
Waiting in queues
Lifts
Enclosed spaces (e.g. tunnels)
Large rooms (lobbies)
Driving or riding in a car (e.g. in a traffic jam)
Walking on the street
Fields, courtyards
High places, bridges
Travelling away from home
Staying at home alone

1.4 **Presumption of organic illness**

Individuals with panic disorder display characteristic concerns or attributions about the implications or consequences of the panic attacks (Box 1.2). Some fear that the attacks indicate the presence of an undiagnosed, life-threatening illness (e.g. a myocardial infarction, a stroke, a brain tumour, or a seizure disorder). Others fear that the panic attacks are an indication that they are 'going crazy' or losing control. Therefore, they frequently present to hospital emergency departments, or have the tendency to undergo repeated medical investigations. Despite repeated reassurance by physicians that all tests were negative, they may remain frightened and unconvinced that they do not have a life-threatening illness. Sometimes, these patients refuse treatment by psychiatrists or psychologists.

In some cases, patients assume the cause to be organic disease only for the time of a panic attack. After the anxiety symptoms fade out, insight into the essentially psychological nature of the condition returns.

Even those patients who have insight into the psychological origin of panic disorder may still believe panic attacks could be harmful to their health (e.g. tachycardia could cause myocardial infarction, or feared collapses could cause accidents).

1.5 **Comorbidity**

Panic disorder complicated by other psychiatric conditions is more common than panic disorder alone. The presence of comorbidity results in more severe anxiety and depressive symptoms, a higher rate of suicide attempts, a higher frequency of other comorbid conditions, and a poorer response and adherence with treatment than in patients with panic disorder alone (Lecrubier, 1998).

Although comorbidity of any type may occur in either men or women with panic disorder, there is a tendency towards higher comorbidity rates in women for certain

Box 1.2 **Clinical example**

The following example represents a typical case of panic disorder with agoraphobia:

Mrs Sandra S., aged 36 years, started to have panic attacks after giving birth to her child 5 years previously. During the attacks, which lasted for approximately half an hour, she suffered from a fast and irregular heart beat, trembling, dizziness, the feeling that she could faint at any moment, numb feelings in her face and on her left body side, and fear of dying. Several times, she was referred to emergency treatments in a hospital, where a complete check-up did not reveal any irregularities. Very often, she was on sick leave from work due to her anxiety attacks. Around 6 months after the first attacks, she developed agoraphobia in crowded spaces. As a consequence, she tended to avoid going to parties, restaurants, shopping malls or cinemas. Her general practitioner started to treat her with St John's wort tablets and homoeopathic formulations, which did not change the course of illness. She was referred to a psychosomatic unit where she had individual and group psychotherapy for 3 months. Whilst there, she reported some relief in panic symptoms, but no complete remission. Soon after discharge, her symptoms reappeared. After 2 years of severe panic disorder, she was referred to the University Department clinic for anxiety disorders. She underwent treatment with an SSRI (escitalopram 20 mg/day), which showed efficacy after 3 weeks. Initial jitteriness disappeared after 10 days. Moreover, the patient also undertook 20 sessions of individual, ambulatory cognitive behavioural therapy, which involved therapist-guided exposure to crowded places. The patient was in stable remission and could resume work.

4

disorders—specific phobia, generalized anxiety disorder (GAD), bipolar disorder, and dysthymia. Men have a tendency for higher comorbidity rates for social anxiety disorder and hypochondriasis, and are significantly more likely to have a history of past alcohol dependence or abuse.

1.5.1 **Other anxiety disorders**

In a large representative survey, 94% of patients with panic disorder and agoraphobia also had another anxiety disorder. Specific phobia was the most prevalent condition (75%), followed by social phobia (67%) and post-traumatic stress disorder (40%). The overlap with obsessive–compulsive disorder (20%) and GAD (15%) was less frequent, but still substantial (Kessler et al, 2006). However, in clinical practice, the most prominent anxiety syndrome can often be identified in an individual patient, despite the high overlap among the anxiety disorders.

1.5.2 **Depression**

There is a strong association between panic disorder and depression. Panic disorder and depression may have common neurobiological and genetic origins. This explains why some patients suffering from (pure) panic disorder may develop (pure) major depression later in their life, or vice versa. However, some patients develop 'secondary depression' as a consequence of 'demoralization' due to recurrent panic attacks, anticipatory anxiety, and the restrictions in quality of life due to avoidance of feared situations. These patients do not necessarily fulfil the criteria for major depression. Secondary depression should improve along with the remission of panic symptoms.

Patients with anxious depression sometimes suffer from additional panic attacks and agoraphobic avoidance, but in this case depressive symptoms usually predominate. When patients aged 60 years or more without a history of panic disorder present with panic attacks, they should be monitored closely for symptoms of depression, as panic disorder rarely occurs in this age group.

1.5.3 Suicidality

Panic disorder and panic attacks are associated with an elevated risk of suicidal idea-tion. In one study, 31% of patients with panic disorder reported suicidal thoughts (Cox et al, 1994). In a clinical sample, a high rate of 42% of suicide attempts was reported (Lépine et al, 1993). However, when controlling for comorbid conditions known to increase suicide risk, panic disorder was not associated with an increased risk of suicide attempts (Hornig and McNally, 1995). The high rate of suicide attempts is not always accompanied by a higher rate of completed suicide. In a psychological autopsy study of completed suicides, panic disorder, and non-comorbid panic disorder in particular, appeared to be rare (Henriksson et al, 1996). It seems that the comorbid conditions of depression, alcohol abuse, or personality disorders are the main risk factors associated with the risk of death from suicide attempts in patients with panic disorder.

1.5.4 Substance abuse

People with panic disorder are more likely to abuse alcohol and sedative hypnotics than the general population, presumably due to the anxiolytic properties of these sub-stances. Any substance disorder occurred in 38% of patients with panic disorder and agoraphobia (Kessler et al, 2006). A significant familial transmission contributes to the co-occurrence (Cosci et al, 2007). When panic disorder is compounded by substance abuse, treatment is often more challenging.

1.5.5 Personality disorders and other psychiatric conditions

Panic disorder is often comorbid with personality disorder. In particular, patients with borderline personality disorder frequently suffer from panic attacks. However, the clinical picture of this personality disorder can be easily differentiated in most cases by monitoring for other more characteristic features, for example, impulse control disor-der, self-injury, unsteady personal relationships, eating disorders, and other symptoms. Borderline features may negatively influence treatment response (Marchesi et al, 2006). Other disorders associated with panic disorder include attention-deficit/hyperactivity disorder (ADHD) or other impulse-control disorders.

1.6 Differential diagnosis

1.6.1 Other psychiatric disorders

Due to the presence of non-specific somatic symptoms, when establishing the diag-nosis of panic disorder, physicians must consider other mental disorders or medical conditions that may mimic panic attacks.

Panic attacks may occur in other anxiety disorders (Table 1.1). Some patients with social anxiety disorder (SAD) suffer from attack-like symptoms in certain feared social or performance situations. However, they usually do not have fear of dying during the attacks and worry less about their physical symptoms than about the social consequences of the special situation. Patients with SAD also avoid crowds, but not because the fear of suffocation or fainting in the crowd, but because of their fears that they might be scrutinized and evaluated negatively by others.

Patients with GAD can suffer from the same anxiety symptoms that occur during a panic attack, like tachycardia, trembling, sweating, gastrointestinal problems, and others, but these symptoms do not occur all at the same time in the form of attack-like anxiety, but are usually present in various combinations for many hours or even for the whole day. While patients with panic disorder are more worried about their own health, GAD patients tend to worry about mishaps or accidents that might happen to their close relatives or friends.

As in patients with agoraphobia, people with specific phobia may be afraid of heights: but in agoraphobia, this is only one of several fears, whereas in specific phobia, fear is typically restricted to only this phobia.

When patients present with symptoms of both depression and panic disorder, differential diagnosis may be a challenging task. The order of appearance of the symptoms, the patient's history, the family history, and the age of the patient at time of occurrence

Table 1.1 Differential diagnosis of panic disorder: Other psychiatric disorders		
Disorder	Features	Differentiating features
Generalized anxiety disorder (GAD)	Anxiety symptoms like palpitations, tremor, shortness of breath etc.	No attack-like anxiety, like in panic disorder. In GAD, patients are more worried about the health of relatives, while in PD, patients are worried about their own health
Social anxiety disorder (SAD)	Fear in crowds or social gatherings	In agoraphobia fear of having a panic attack in a crowd; in SAD, fear of being scrutinized by others
	Panic attacks	Panic attacks in SAD are restricted to social situations and rarely occur when alone (unless when anticipating a social situation)
Specific phobia	Fear of heights, lifts, driving, flying, public transportation, enclosed places	In specific phobia, fear is restricted to single situations
Obsessive–compulsive disorder (OCD)	Panic attacks	Panic cued by thoughts of or exposure to the object or situation related to an obsession (e.g., exposure to dirt in a patient with an obsession about contamination)
Post-traumatic stress disorder	Panic attacks	Panic attacks cued by stimuli recalling the traumatic event
Depression	Fear of going out in public	In depression, avoidance of gatherings with other people is due to anhedonia
Somatoform disorders	Fear of having severe medical disorders; patients can hardly be convinced that they are physically healthy	Frequently changing clinical picture in somatoform disorders, but no anxiety attacks. Joint and muscle pain, headache and other pain syndromes

of the symptoms have to be taken into account in the differential diagnosis. It may be helpful to simply ask the patient, which of depression or panic is in the foreground, as in most cases, patients have a clear opinion on which symptom complex is more prominent. As mentioned previously, in elderly patients, anxious depression is the more likely diagnosis, as panic disorder is rare in this age group.

Patients with panic disorder often have hypochondriacal beliefs that they might suffer from severe medical illnesses. Therefore, the differentiation from somatoform disorders may sometimes be difficult. Patients with somatization disorder may also present with anxiety symptoms, but usually do not report complete panic attacks. They present with various frequently changing physical complaints, some of which resemble anxiety symptoms (e.g. tachycardia, tremor, or dyspnoea), while others are not typical for anxiety disorders (e.g. joint and muscle pain or headaches). These patients find it hard to be convinced that their symptoms have no organic cause. Like panic patients, they often demand additional investigations. However, patients with panic disorders usually have more insight into the psychological causation of their symptoms.

1.6.2 **Non-psychiatric disorders**

A number of medical conditions have to be excluded before a diagnosis of panic disorder can be made (Table 1.2). Routine diagnostic measures that should be performed in patients presenting with anxiety symptoms are summarized in Table 1.3. A physician should make concerted efforts to monitor patients for other medical conditions before diagnosing panic disorder. However, if patients still remain unconvinced that they are physically healthy and demand more medical investigations in spite of thorough medical examinations, the physician should refrain from performing unnecessary examinations and try to explain that further investigations are unnecessary.

1.6.2.1 *Heart disease*

Many of the symptoms of panic disorder are also cardinal features of cardiovascular diseases. Patients with panic disorder may initially present to emergency care facilities complaining of acute chest pain or other cardiovascular symptoms. Approximately one-quarter of patients who present to physicians for treatment of chest pain have panic disorder (Huffman et al, 2002). Such patients are then often submitted to costly, invasive cardiac testing procedures. It was estimated that these patients account for at least one third of those who undergo angiography for the evaluation of chest pain and are subsequently found to have normal coronary arteries (Mukerji et al, 1993).

Panic attacks may also occur in patients with coronary artery disease, but it is unclear whether panic disorder confers additional risk for or exacerbates cardiac disorders (Fleet et al, 2000). Although many patients with panic disorder are misdiagnosed as 'cardiac cases', there is some evidence that panic disorder may be linked with cardiovascular disease: patients with panic disorder were observed to have nearly a two-fold increased risk for coronary heart disease (Gomez-Caminero et al, 2005).

A higher rate of mitral valve prolapse in patients with panic disorder has been reported (Katerndahl, 1993). However, it has been assumed that the mitral valve prolapse associated with panic disorder is a benign variant, which does not require specific treatment. In a study with panic patients, the severity of mitral valve prolapse was mild; nearly all of the cases were silent, without cardiac murmur, and there was no problem with left ventricular function (Hamada et al, 1998).

Table 1.2 Differential diagnosis of panic disorder: medical conditions that can mimic panic attacks

Differential diagnosis	Symptoms that mimic panic attacks	Distinguishing symptoms
Cardiac arrhythmias	Irregular heartbeat	ECG
Angina pectoris	Chest pain, anxiety, dyspnoea	Exercise ECG, nitroglycerine test
Myocardial infarction	Sudden chest pain (typically radiating to the left arm), dyspnoea, palpitations, sweating, anxiety (sense of impending doom)	ECG, blood tests
Syncope	Dizziness, fainting, nausea	Portable ECG, tilt table test
Pulmonary embolism	Dyspnoea, feeling of choking, chest pain	Cough, haemoptysis, pleural rub, cyanosis, collapse, circulatory instability
Asthma	Dyspnoea, choking, smothering sensations, chest pain	Inspiration difficulties in panic disorder, expiration problems in asthma
Vestibular dysfunctions	Dizziness, somnolence, nausea, vomiting, anxiety	Caloric reflex test, electro-nystagmography, videonystagmography, rotation tests
Seizure disorders	Anxiety, derealization, depersonalization, sweating, blushing, dyspnoea, hyperventilation, tachycardia, nausea	Video-EEG
Migraine	Headache, paraesthesias, nausea	Severe headache, photophobia, flickering lights, hyperacusis
Multiple sclerosis	Dizziness, paraesthesias	CSF, MRT, evoked potentials
Hypoglycaemia	Tachycardia, tremor, anxiety, sweating, dizziness, gastrointestinal complaints	Blood glucose levels
Hyperthyroidism	Anxiety, tachycardia, palpitations, sweating, dyspnoea, diarrhoea	Thyroid-stimulating hormone (TSH)
Hyperkalaemia	Palpitations, arrhythmia, paraesthesias	Potassium concentration
Acute porphyria	Anxiety, gastrointestinal discomfort, paraesthesias, tachycardia, arrhythmia, agitation, depression	Spectroscopy, biochemical analysis of blood, urine, and stool
Insulinoma	Tremor, sweating, syncope, palpitations, tachycardia, sweating, anxiety, nausea	Glucose, insulin, C-peptide
Carcinoid syndrome	Diarrhoea, respiratory distress	5-hydroxy-indol-acetic acid, chromogranin A
Phaeochromocytoma	Anxiety, tachycardia, hypertension, tremor, headache, sweating, hot flushes	Catecholamines and metanephrines in plasma, clonidine suppression test

CSF, cerebrospinal fluid; ECG, electrocardiograph; EEG, electroencephalogram; MRT, magnetic resonance tomography

Table 1.3 Potential diagnostic evaluations in patients with panic disorder	
Internal medicine	Clinical examination, blood pressure, heart rate, blood tests, ECG, exercise ECG, 24-hour ECG, 24-hour blood pressure, chest X-ray, echocardiography
Neurology	EEG, MRT, CSF, Doppler sonography
Otolaryngology	Caloric reflex test, electronystagmography, videonystagmography, rotation tests

CSF, cerebrospinal fluid; ECG, electrocardiograph; EEG, electroencephalogram; MRT

1.6.2.2 *Pulmonary disease*

The majority of panic disorder patients experience breathing-related problems. In the case of acute panic symptoms, some patients may have to be monitored for pulmonary embolism, a potentially lethal condition. Panic disorder also shares a number of symptoms with asthma, such as dyspnoea, choking, sensations of being smothered, and chest pain. However, panic patients report inspiration difficulties, while asthma is characterized by expiration problems. More than one in five individuals with asthma report having experienced panic attacks (Carr et al, 1996).

1.7 **Course**

Panic disorder typically begins between late adolescence and the mid-30s: onset after age 45 years is unusual. The median age at onset is 24 years (Kessler et al, 2005a). The prevalence of panic disorder is greatest in the 25–44-year age group. After the age of around 45, symptoms slowly diminish until they disappear completely in most patients. Recurrent attacks may occur for years. The course is usually chronic, but symptoms usually wax and wane in severity. Some individuals may have episodic outbreaks with years of intervening full or partial remission, whereas others may have continuous severe symptomatology. In patients presenting with agoraphobia, this develops about half a year on average after the first panic attacks.

Typically, there is a substantial period between initial onset and presentation for treatment. This is not only due to the problem of under-diagnosing in primary care, but also to the tendency of patients to assume the presence of physical illness, rather than a psychiatric disorder. Naturalistic follow-up studies of individuals treated in tertiary care settings (which may select for a poor-prognosis group) suggest that, at 6–10 years post-treatment, about 30% of individuals are well, 40–50% are improved but symptomatic, and the remaining 20–30% have symptoms that are the same or slightly worse.

1.8 **Prevalence**

A general population survey, the United States NCS (National Comorbidity Survey—Replication) has estimated the lifetime prevalence to be 6% for panic disorder and 1.6% for agoraphobia without panic disorder, the 12-months prevalence rates being 2.7% and 0.8% (Kessler et al, 2005a, b). Apparently, there has been no substantial change in prevalence rates since the first survey conducted between 1990 and 1992 and the second conducted from 2001 to 2003 (Kessler et al, 2005c). It is estimated that 22% of the population experience at least one panic attack during their life without meeting full diagnostic criteria for panic disorder (Kessler et al, 2006).

The disorder is at least twice as common in women than in men (Wittchen et al, 1992). Panic disorder has been found in epidemiological studies throughout the world. In some cultures, panic attacks may involve intense fear of witchcraft or magic. Moreover, a number of 'culture-bound syndromes' may be related to panic disorder.

Among the major anxiety disorders, panic disorder with or without agoraphobia (12-months prevalence 3.5%) is less frequent than social anxiety disorder (6.8%) and approximately as common as generalized anxiety disorder (3.1%). In clinical settings, however, panic disorder is by far the most prevalent disorder, probably due to the high health care utilization in this group. In a University Anxiety Disorders Outpatient Unit, 52% of the patients with anxiety disorders had panic disorder, while 10.3% of the sample, had sad and 7.5% had GAD.

1.9 **Quality of life and health care utilization**

Some individuals with recurrent panic attacks make significant changes in their behaviour (e.g. retire from social activities, quit a job, or avoid physical exertion) in response to the attacks. The often chronic course of panic disorder is associated with quality-of-life impairment, including substance abuse, an increased likelihood of suicide attempts, impaired social and marital functioning, lower educational achievement, lower work productivity due to frequent sick leave or early retirement, and a higher likelihood of unemployment (Ettigi et al, 1997).

Patients with panic disorder are particularly high users of healthcare services. Most patients with panic disorder obtained lifetime treatment for psychiatric problems (96.1% among those with agoraphobia and 84.8% without). Studies suggest that approximately one-third of patients with panic disorder visit three or more healthcare specialists per year. One study revealed that almost one-fifth of patients with panic disorder had attended a general hospital emergency department and that 1 in 10 had been hospitalized at some point for anxiety complaints (Swinson et al, 1992).

Cardiologists, neurologists, otolaryngologists, obstetrician–gynaecologists, and urologists are also seen more frequently by people with panic disorder than by people with other psychiatric disorders (Kennedy and Schwab, 1997). The primary reason for referral to non-psychiatrist specialists is probably not the underdiagnosis by GPs due to a lack of specific psychiatric knowledge or to a general underestimation of psychiatric problems, but rather may lie in the disorder itself, as it is associated with the tendency to assume the presence of a medical illness rather than a psychiatric disorder. The search for medical causes of the symptoms may distract both physicians and patients from the real problem.

The total direct costs of healthcare use and indirect costs of lost productivity are considerable and are greater than for other mental disorders (Batelaan et al, 2007). The costs of non-diagnosis are usually overlooked when estimating the global costs of panic disorder.

Though patients suffering from panic disorder exhibit high medical help-seeking, only approximately half of the patients obtain treatment consistent with basic treatment guidelines (Kessler et al, 2006).

1.10 **Assessment**

The diagnosis of panic disorder should be made by using the current versions of the classification systems (International Classification of Diseases, ICD, and DSM). For assessing severity of panic disorder and agoraphobia, a number of rating scales are available. In general practice, rating scales are not commonly used, due to time limitations. However, in psychiatric clinics, they should be used to objectively monitor treatment progress. For research purposes and in clinical trials the use of these scales is essential.

Two scales are mainly used in the assessment of severity in panic disorder. The Panic and Agoraphobia Scale (P&A) (Bandelow, 1999)(see Appendix 2) was developed in 1993, and has been used in a number of randomized controlled trials. A similar scale was developed in the US, the Panic Disorder Severity Scale (Shear et al, 1997). The use of either of these two scales has been recommended by the European Medicines Agency for use in panic disorder treatment studies (EMA, 2005).

The severity of panic disorder should not only be measured by counting the number of panic attacks. Using panic frequency as an outcome measure is tempting: it appears to be an exact measure when compared to relatively non-specific rating scale items such as 'moderate' or 'severe anxiety'. However, the number of attacks is an insufficient measure—as would be counting the number of times that a depressed patients cries instead of employing a validated depression scale. Panic attacks are not the only feature of panic disorder influencing severity and impacting on quality of life. A patient might have a score of zero on panic frequency and therefore appear to be in remission, but might still have marked and disabling agoraphobia: by contrast, another patient may have very infrequent panic attacks, but suffer from severe anticipatory anxiety. Other patients are concerned that their symptoms are not due to a psychological but to an internal or neurological disease, such as coronary heart disease or a brain tumour. They may live in constant fear of being wrongly diagnosed. Five principal symptom domains of panic disorder have been identified and are shown in Box 1.3.

One advantage of the P&A scale is that it is subdivided into five subscales, each representing a key feature of panic disorder that can be analysed separately. Moreover the panic attack domain not only evaluates the frequency of attacks, but also their severity and duration. Although the P&A scale is not a diagnostic instrument, the patient-rated version may be used as a time-saving screening tool for assessing panic symptomatology.

In addition to the present symptoms, the routine assessment for patients suspected of having panic disorder should also include the following items:

- Onset of symptoms (present episode, earlier episodes)
- Patient history (other psychiatric disorders, childhood experiences, separation anxiety during childhood, etc.)
- Family history (other family members with panic disorder, etc.)
- Impact on quality of life (family relationships, job situation, social integration)
- Previous treatments and their efficacy (previous drug treatments, dosage, duration of intake, psychological and 'alternative' treatments).

> ## Box 1.3 Five principal symptom domains of panic disorder
>
> • Panic attacks (frequency, severity, duration)
> • Agoraphobic avoidance
> • Anticipatory anxiety
> • Functional disability (including work, social, and family function)
> • Assumption of somatic disorders

References and further reading

APA (2000) *Diagnostic and Statistical Manual of Mental Disorders, Fourth Edition, Text Revision (DSM-IV-TR®)* American Psychiatric Press, Washington, DC.

Bandelow B (1999). *Panic and Agoraphobia Scale (PAS)*. Hogrefe & Huber Publishers, Göttingen/Bern/Toronto/Seattle.

Batelaan N, Smit F, de Graaf R, van Balkom A, Vollebergh W, Beekman A (2007). Economic costs of full-blown and subthreshold panic disorder. *J Affect Disord* **104**: 127–36.

Carr RE, Lehrer PM, Hochron SM, Jackson A (1996). Effect of psychological stress on airway impedance in individuals with asthma and panic disorder. *J Abnorm Psychol* **105**: 137–41.

Cosci F, Schruers KR, Abrams K, Griez EJ (2007). Alcohol use disorders and panic disorder: a review of the evidence of a direct relationship. *J Clin Psychiatry* **68**: 874–80.

Cox BJ, Direnfeld DM, Swinson RP, Norton GR (1994). Suicidal ideation and suicide attempts in panic disorder and social phobia. *Am J Psychiatry* **151**: 882–7.

EMA (2005). European Medicines Agency. Committee for Medicinal Products for Human Use (CHMP). Guideline on Clinical Investigation of Medicinal Products Indicated for the Treatment of Panic Disorder. http://www.ema.europa.eu/docs/en_GB/document_library/Scientific_guideline/2009/09/WC500003511.pdf (accessed 13 May 2013).

Ettigi P, Meyerhoff AS, Chirban JT, Jacobs RJ, Wilson RR (1997). The quality of life and employ-ment in panic disorder. *J Nerv Ment Dis* **185**: 368–72.

Fleet R, Lavoie K, Beitman BD (2000). Is panic disorder associated with coronary artery disease? A critical review of the literature. *J Psychosom Res* **48**: 347–56.

Gomez-Caminero A, Blumentals WA, Russo LJ, Brown RR, Castilla-Puentes R (2005). Does panic disorder increase the risk of coronary heart disease? A cohort study of a national managed care database. *Psychosom Med* **67**: 688–91.

Hamada T, Koshino Y, Misawa T, Isaki K, Gejyo F (1998). Mitral valve prolapse and autonomic function in panic disorder. *Acta Psychiatr Scand* **97**: 139–43.

Henriksson MM, Isometsa ET, Kuoppasalmi KI, Heikkinen ME, Marttunen MJ, Lonnqvist JK (1996). Panic disorder in completed suicide. *J Clin Psychiatry* **57**: 275–81.

Hornig CD, McNally RJ (1995). Panic disorder and suicide attempt. A reanalysis of data from the Epidemiologic Catchment Area study. *Br J Psychiatry* **167**: 76–9.

Huffman JC, Pollack MH, Stern TA (2002). Panic Disorder and Chest Pain: Mechanisms, Morbidity, and Management. *Prim Care Companion J Clin Psychiatry* **4**: 54–62.

Katerndahl DA (1993). Panic and prolapse. Meta-analysis. *J Nerv Ment Dis* **181**: 539–44.

Kennedy BL, Schwab JJ (1997). Utilization of medical specialists by anxiety disorder patients. *Psychosomatics* **38**: 109–12.

Kessler RC, Berglund P, Demler O, Jin R, Merikangas KR, Walters EE (2005a). Lifetime preva-lence and age-of-onset distributions of DSM-IV disorders in the National Comorbidity Survey Replication. *Arch Gen Psychiatry* **62**: 593–602.

Kessler RC, Chiu WT, Demler O, Merikangas KR, Walters EE (2005b). Prevalence, severity, and comorbidity of 12-month DSM-IV disorders in the National Comorbidity Survey Replication. *Arch Gen Psychiatry* **62**: 617–27.

Kessler RC, Demler O, Frank RG, Olfson M, Pincus HA, Walters EE, Wang P, Wells KB, Zaslavsky AM (2005c). Prevalence and treatment of mental disorders, 1990 to 2003. *N Engl J Med* **352**: 2515–23.

Kessler RC, Chiu WT, Jin R, Ruscio AM, Shear K, Walters EE (2006). The epidemiology of panic attacks, panic disorder, and agoraphobia in the National Comorbidity Survey Replication. *Arch Gen Psychiatry* **63**: 415–24.

Lecrubier Y (1998). The impact of comorbidity on the treatment of panic disorder. *J Clin Psychiatry* **59** (Suppl 8): 11–4; discussion 15–6.

Lépine JP, Chignon JM, Teherani M (1993). Suicide attempts in patients with panic disorder. *Arch Gen Psychiatry* **50**: 144–9.

Marchesi C, De Panfilis C, Cantoni A, Fonto S, Giannelli MR, Maggini C (2006). Personality disorders and response to medication treatment in panic disorder: a 1-year naturalistic study. *Prog Neuropsychopharmacol Biol Psychiatry* **30**: 1240–5.

Mukerji V, Beitman BD, Alpert MA (1993). Chest pain and angiographically normal coronary arteries. Implications for treatment. *Tex Heart Inst J* **20**: 170–9.

Shear MK, Brown TA, Barlow DH, Money R, Sholomskas DE, Woods SW, Gorman JM, Papp LA (1997). Multicenter collaborative panic disorder severity scale. *Am J Psychiatry* **154**: 1571–5.

Swinson RP, Cox BJ, Woszczyna CB (1992). Use of medical services and treatment for panic disorder with agoraphobia and for social phobia. *Can Med Assoc J* **147**: 878–83.

Wittchen HU, Essau CA, von Zerssen D, Krieg JC, Zaudig M (1992). Lifetime and six-month prevalence of mental disorders in the Munich Follow-Up Study. *Eur Arch Psychiatry Clin Neurosci* **241**: 247–58.

Chapter 2

Aetiology

Key points

- The aetiology of panic disorder is multifactorial, including environmental, genetic, and neurobiological factors.
- Among environmental factors, severe early traumatic life events (e.g. separation from parents, sexual abuse) have been associated with panic disorder, while parental rearing styles seem to have only a minor role.
- Panic disorder has a strong genetic component with an interaction of multiple risk genes, each with only a minor individual effect
- Evidence for neurobiological dysfunctions in panic disorder is derived from the efficacy of certain drugs and from comparisons of panic patients to healthy controls. Among other hypotheses, dysfunctions of serotonergic neurotransmission may play a role in the aetiology of panic disorder.

2.1 **Introduction**

Anxiety symptoms are characterized by normal physiological reactions that can be explained by 'fight or flight' situations that help the organism to survive. An animal threatened by another dangerous animal has to decide to either run away or to struggle for its life. Therefore, the heartbeat, blood pressure, and breathing frequency is increased physiologically, in order to prepare the body for fast running or fierce fighting. The eyes are opened wide and all senses are set to high attention. The blood is diverted into the muscles in preparation for a burst of emergency action, resulting in paleness and numbing feelings in the face or fingers. All symptoms of a panic attack can be explained by a survival function of the body. Even the 'goose-flesh skin' that we may experience in a feared situation may be explained by a rudimentary body function seen in furry animals—the piloerection may make the animal look bigger.

When a danger is perceived, two pathways in the brain are activated—sometimes understood as the 'low road' and the 'high road'. The first is a fast, unconscious, primitive, and innate reaction, occurring within thousandths of seconds. Without this emergency reaction, we could be dead before we are able to analyse the danger situation. The second reaction is rather slow, conscious, intelligent, and rational. It collects detailed and specific information about the threat.

Anxiety and fear are controlled by an 'anxiety network', an association of various brain structures, which has been described by LeDoux et al (1990), Gorman et al. (2000), Charney and Bremner (1999), and others. In Fig. 2.1, the fear circuits of the brain are described. Due to space limits, the description is simplified.

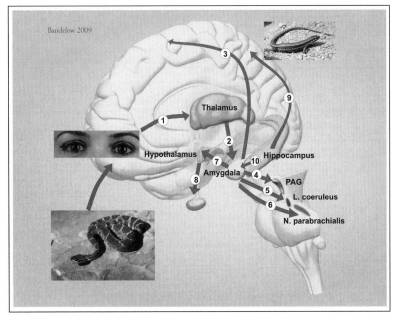

Figure 2.1 Fear circuits in the brain. © Borwin Bandelow 2009

Notes:

1. The thalamus collects information about fear-eliciting stimuli from all senses, e.g. seeing a snake, hearing the roar of a tiger, or smelling a fire. Also, threatening inputs from the body are analysed, e.g. chest pain, increased heartbeat or information about the lack of oxygen. The thalamus initiates two strategies: (a) a fast, but unspecific emergency response, and (b) a slower, but precise analysis of the situation.

2. In the fast response strategy, the thalamus 'analyses' the situation to determine whether it corresponds to an innate instinctual fear, by scanning the fear situation and matching it up with primitive pictures of snakes, spiders, or other dangers, that are stored in a special inborn 'survival memory'. The amygdala is alerted and initiates a number of reactions:

3. By informing motor centres, a quick motor reaction is initiated (e.g. a fast step backwards).

4. In the periaqueductal grey matter, freezing is initiated in animals, or fear of death in humans.

5. In the locus coeruleus, blood pressure and heart rate are increased.

6. In the nucleus parabrachialis, breathing frequency is increased.

7. In the hypothalamus, the sympathetic nervous system is activated.

8. Also in the hypothalamus, the HPA axis is activated, leading to in release of CRH, which acts on the pituitary gland.

9. In the slow response strategy, the hippocampus analyses the threat situation by retrieving detailed information from all available memory sources, including theoretical knowledge about spiders, or the recall of previous unpleasant experiences. It may come to the conclusion that the slithering shape that was mistaken for a snake by the primitive anxiety system turns out to be a harmless lizard.

10. The amygdala is informed that the threatening situation is harmless and that the bodily reaction can be scaled down.

However, a patient experiencing panic symptoms has no obvious explanation for the changes in the body, as he or she is not in a fight or flight situation, but perhaps sitting in front of the television set. As a logical consequence, the patient assumes there is a terrible malfunction of the body that requires help by a physician.

It might be hypothesized that there is a centre somewhere in the brain that monitors the body for malfunctions of the heart or other organs. For example, when we climb up a mountain, this centre warns us that we have to take a break from time to time in order not to overstress our body. In panic disorder, this centre seems to be oversensitive, warning us of a non-existing danger.

2.2 Environmental factors

The early psychoanalytic literature attributed the origin of anxiety disorders to two major causes: to early traumatic life events, such as the death of the mother or sexual abuse during childhood; or to certain parental attitudes or child-rearing styles, such as neglecting or controlling behaviour of the mother. The literature was not specific to what kind of trauma, as it was assumed that nearly all kinds of psychological disturbances could have their origin in various kinds of traumas. However, these possible aetiological factors have not been investigated systematically.

In a first large-scale retrospective study in patients with panic disorder (Bandelow et al, 2002), the frequency of reports of some traumatic childhood experiences was significantly different between patients and controls: including death of father, separation from parents, childhood illness, parents' alcohol abuse, violence in the family, sexual abuse, and other factors. Only one-third of panic patients, but two-thirds of the controls did not report any severe traumatic events at all. However, in a logistic regression model, a family history of anxiety disorders was a much stronger predictor than was severe traumatic events during childhood.

Compared to controls, patients with panic disorder described the attitude of their parents as more restricting and providing less loving care and attention than healthy controls. However, in the logistic regression model, this association seemed to be due to other confounding factors. According to this study, the contribution of unfavourable parental rearing styles was very small. There is an association between separation anxiety disorder in childhood and adult panic disorder. However, this was not correlated with actual separation experiences in childhood (Bandelow et al, 2001).

2.2.1 Stressful life events

Panic disorder is often preceded by stressful life events (Faravelli et al, 1985). Loss or disruption of important interpersonal relationships (e.g. leaving home to live on one's own, separation, or divorce) is associated with the exacerbation of panic disorder. Also, severe illnesses in close relatives, such as a myocardial infarction, may initiate an episode of panic attacks. However, it does not seem probable that stressful life events in adulthood can act as the sole aetiological factor in panic disorder. Rather, an exacerbation of existing panic disorder can be triggered by stressful life events in some vulnerable patients. The majority of patients do not report relevant stress events before the onset or exacerbation of their anxiety disorder. Whereas some panic attacks are directly triggered by a stress situation, for example a major argument with a spouse, a financial loss, or illness of a close relative, this is more the exception than the rule. Most panic attacks occur in harmless situations, such as when reading a book or walking in a shopping mall. Some patients report that a first panic attack was a stressful life event itself, being the cause for all following panic attacks.

2.2.2 Psychodynamic approaches

One of the earliest psychological models of pathological anxiety was the one developed by Sigmund Freud (Freud, 1964). During his life, Freud changed his theories about anxiety. In his 'First Anxiety Theory', he assumed that panic attacks might occur when sexual desires could not be satisfied, for example in couples before their marriage. In a later theory, he claimed that anxiety occurred when unconscious and forbidden sexual desires of the Ego were detected by the Superego and punished by inducing anxiety symptoms.

Freud's theories underwent various modifications, and today, there is no uniform homogeneous or generally accepted psychoanalytic theory for panic disorder. In general, there is a tendency in psychodynamic approaches to find a different explanation for anxiety symptoms for each patient rather than to develop a comprehensive model that applies to the majority of panic sufferers. This has the advantage that every patient is seen as an individual, but does not facilitate the development of universally applicable theories.

According to a current psychoanalytic theory (Busch et al, 1999), panic symptoms carry psychological meanings, and psychodynamic psychotherapy works to uncover unconscious meanings to achieve relief. From early life, individuals prone to panic struggle with feelings of inadequacy and a sense of being dependent on caretakers to provide safety. A repetition of this vicious cycle is triggered in adulthood when fantasies or experiences of disruption in attachments occur, frequently triggered by meaningful life events. The defence mechanisms of 'reaction formation' and 'undoing' represent efforts to deny anger and make attachments closer through compensatory positive feelings. However, because of angry feelings that are at least partly unconscious, these defences ultimately fail to modulate the experienced threat to attachment—leading to the onset of panic. Some patients report a frightening or arousing inherent excitement associated with the attacks, often closely tied to presumed sadomasochistic sexual fantasies. Panic attacks can serve a self-punitive function with which patients unconsciously atone for guilty transgressions.

Psychoanalytic theories, however, are largely based on individual case reports and theoretical considerations and have not undergone formal examination by means of empirical investigations. The lack of controlled efficacy studies also hampers the recognition of psychoanalytic treatment as a standard therapy for anxiety disorders.

2.2.3 Learning theories

According to cognitive theories of panic disorder, patients with panic attacks have an enduring tendency to misinterpret benign bodily sensations as indications of an immediately impending physical catastrophe. For example, palpitations and chest pain may be interpreted as evidence of an imminent myocardial infarction. A vicious circle is started, in which initial fear symptoms such as palpitations lead to further anxiety symptoms such as dyspnoea, which again trigger other physiological fear reactions, eventually culminating in a full-blown panic attack. According to this cognitive model, agoraphobia also is a result of a learning process. When a panic attack occurs in a harmless situation, this situation serves as a conditioned stimulus. As a consequence, the patient tries to avoid this situation in the future. For example, a man has drunk a strong cup of coffee. Later, he uses a lift, where he experiences tachycardia due to the caffeine effects. Then, he falsely associates his tachycardia with the lift situation. His fear increases and more panic symptoms occur, eventually resulting in the picture of a complete panic attack. As a consequence, he avoids lifts in the future.

This theory of the 'vicious circle' of panic attacks is not undisputed. Most patients report that all the symptoms of a panic attack occur simultaneously, not one after the other, which is in accordance to the theory that these attacks are a 'fight or flight' reaction. Panic attacks also can occur during non-rapid eye movement (NREM) sleep, a state with minimal cognitive activity (Mellman and Uhde, 1990).

Earlier versions of behavioural theories did not consider that there are certain situations that are more prone to trigger panic attacks than others. Seligman developed the 'preparedness theory', which hypothesises that phobic fears are associated more easily with certain situations or objects that the individual is prepared for (Seligman, 1971). For example, simple phobias may be seen as reminiscent of earlier instinctive fears. Fears of spiders and snakes were vital to survive in our ancestors, but are unnecessary today in northern European countries. These fears were genetically transmitted from generation to generation, as they were advantageous in a Darwinian sense by guaranteeing our survival. It would not make sense if snake phobia only developed after a bad experience, because the individual would not have a second chance to take advantage of this learning process after the fatal bite of a poisonous viper.

Agoraphobia does not usually occur as a consequence of traumatic experiences like being trapped in a lift or a tunnel. Agoraphobic fears may be seen as situations that earlier in our evolution were truly dangerous. For example, being trapped in a cave could lead to suffocation or being the prey of a bear; heights were dangerous (and still are); in open fields, the individual was more endangered by wolves or other animals. However, it seems more plausible that agoraphobic situations can better be brought together as situations in which medical help may difficult to obtain. Usually, agoraphobia develops after experiencing some unexpected panic attacks. Also, general medical knowledge about heart attacks or strokes is taken into account by patients when they develop their own explanations about panic attacks. This requires the involvement of higher cognitive functions than for the rudimentary fear of spiders.

The learning theory model of panic disorder has some weaknesses. First, panic symptoms do not seem to appear in a vicious circle one after the other, but mostly all symptoms begin at the same time, according to reports of patients. If the vicious circle of a panic attacks could simply be triggered by one initial anxiety symptom, patients should also have panic attacks in actually dangerous situations, like when closely escaping a car accident, or in other situations that go along with agitation, such as an argument, but this is not the case. Moreover, panic attacks may also occur during NREM sleep, a state in which the brain is in a state of very low activity, so that an initiation by cognitive processes does not seem very likely. In summary, it seems unlikely that panic attacks are merely due to false learning processes. If learning processes play a major role in panic disorder, it would be hard to understand why some patients do not learn, even after hundreds of attacks that did not end in a severe medical condition, that panic attacks themselves are not dangerous.

2.3 Neurobiology

The pathophysiology of panic disorder and the neurobiological basis of panic attacks has been the focus of much research.

2.3.1 Genetics

In first-degree relatives of patients with panic disorder, an up to three-fold increased prevalence of the disorder was observed, which indicates a significant familiality of panic disorder (Maier et al, 1993; Nocon et al, 2008). Twin studies have proposed a considerable contribution of genetic factors to the pathogenesis of panic disorder with heritability estimates ranging from 30–48% for panic disorder and over 50% for agoraphobia (Hettema et al, 2001; Kessler et al, 2005). Segregation analyses, however, have failed to identify a mode of inheritance according to Mendelian patterns; this points to a so-called complex genetic inheritance with an interaction of multiple 'vulnerability' or 'risk genes', each having only a minor individual influence ('oligo-' or 'polygenic' model), with environmental influences (Vieland et al, 1996).

Linkage and association studies have yielded several chromosomal risk loci and risk variants in candidate genes, respectively (for detailed review see: Domschke and Deckert, 2012): potential risk loci for panic disorder have been identified on chromosomes 1p, 4q, 7p, 9q, 11p, 15q and 20p (Crowe et al, 2001; Fyer et al, 2006; Gelernter et al, 2001; Kaabi et al, 2006; Knowles et al, 1998; Thorgeirsson et al, 2003). Association studies revealed the genes coding for catechol-O-methyltransferase (COMT), monoamine oxidase A (MAO_A), the serotonin receptor 1A ($5\text{-}HT_{1A}$), the cholecystokinin B (CCK_B) receptor, the adenosine A2A receptor (ADORA2A), and the neuropeptide S receptor (NPSR1) as the so far most robustly replicated vulnerability genes in panic disorder (Deckert et al, 1998, 1999; Domschke et al, 2004, 2007, 2011; Hamilton et al, 2002, 2004; Hosing et al, 2004; Kennedy et al, 1999; Reif et al, 2012; Rothe et al, 2006; Samochowiec et al, 2004). The first genome-wide association studies, interrogating the entire genome for association using a hypothesis-free approach, point to novel vulnerability genes of panic disorder such as the *TMEM132D* gene, which has been corroborated by functional expression analyses and in an animal model of anxiety (Erhardt et al, 2011).

Gene–environment analyses show a significant impact of adenosine A2A receptor gene variation on anxiety levels after caffeine consumption as a major risk factor for panic disorder (Alsene et al, 2003) and point to early as well as recent negative life events to shape the risk for increased anxiety sensitivity in interaction with the serotonin transporter (5-HTT) and neuropeptide S receptor (NPSR1) genes (Klauke et al, 2011, 2012; Stein et al, 2008). Very recently, epigenetic mechanisms such as DNA methylation have been proposed to potentially mediate the interaction between genetic and environmental factors. The first epigenetic study in panic disorder suggests association of monoamine oxidase A (MAOA) gene DNA hypomethylation with panic disorder particularly in female patients, potentially mediating a detrimental influence of negative life events, while MAOA hypermethylation—possibly conferred by positive life events—has been hypothesized to increase resilience towards the disorder (Domschke et al, 2012).

The molecular genetic analysis of intermediate phenotypes related to panic disorder such as neuronal network activity (Domschke and Dannlowski, 2010) revealed

COMT, 5-HT1A, and NPSR1 variants to confer a distorted corticolimbic activity during anxiety-relevant emotional processing in patients with panic disorder (Domschke et al, 2006, 2008, 2011).

Pharmacogenetic studies investigating the genetically controlled variation in therapy response reported the 5-HTT, 5-HT1A, COMT, and MAOA genes to influence the response to treatment with selective serotonin re-uptake inhibitors (SSRIs) (Perna et al, 2005; Saeki et al, 2009; Yevtushenko et al, 2010) or cognitive-behavioral therapy (Lonsdorf et al, 2010; Reif et al, 2013) in panic disorder.

In summary, there is converging support for a considerable genetic influence on the origin of panic disorder. However, it is still not comprehensively understood how these genes act to confer the disease risk on a functional level. Also, given a complex genetic model of inheritance, a variety of risk genes is assumed to interact with each other as well as with non-genetic risk factors. To date, only a fraction of the risk genes contributing to the development of panic disorder has been identified and not much light has been shed on gene-environment interactions specific for panic disorder. Therefore, the presently identified genetic risk factors are of limited diagnostic or predictive value, which will only change if the entirety of all genetic risk factors interdependent with environmental factors is identified, which is not foreseeable in the near future.

However, genetic research in the field of neuropsychiatry is currently breaking new ground by applying novel methods such as pathway-based analyses and next generation sequencing techniques as well as epigenetic analyses, which are expected to aid in further disentangling the complex-genetic nature of the pathogenesis of panic disorder. Additionally, pharmacogenetic and psychotherapy–genetic studies are likely to unravel some of the variance in the mediation of treatment response in panic disorder. These different roads of research should nourish further biochemical, physiological, or pharmacological efforts in developing innovative drugs for the treatment of panic disorder, preferably in an individually-tailored manner according to genotype.

2.3.2 Animal models

Current knowledge about fear circuits in the brain is largely derived from animal models (LeDoux, 1996). An impressive number of animal models to assess anxiety are available (Fuchs and Flügge, 2006). First, there are models of 'normal' anxiety (e.g. the fear of falling down from a height). These can be separated into models of unconditioned responses (e.g. the elevated plus maze) or those based on conditioned responses (e.g. the Vogel conflict test). Other animal models are paradigms of pathological anxiety. Mutant mice are bred, in which certain genes are deleted that are candidates for anxiety related behaviour: for example, the genes for the 5-HT_{1A} receptor, corticotropin releasing factor receptors, or the γ_2 subunit of the gamma-aminobutyric acid A ($GABA_A$) receptor, a subunit known to be essential in mediating the anxiolytic actions of the benzodiazepines. However, in humans, multiple gene loci are involved in pathological anxiety, and the future may lie in laboratory animals that do not only have one single gene defect, but multiple abnormalities of neurotransmitter circuits that result in anxiety-related behaviour.

However, it must always be kept in mind that fear in laboratory animals is not the same as pathological fear in humans. Laboratory rats are afraid of administered electric shocks or of other male rats, which represent real dangers. In contrast, panic disorder is fear of a non-existing danger, the fear of having a severe medical condition although all organs work well. Brain centres that are responsible for pathological, exaggerated, unrealistic fear may not necessarily be the same as those centres that are handling with real dangers.

2.3.3 Brain imaging

There has been a substantial increase in reports of brain imaging studies in panic disorder. The results of these studies can be hard to interpret, as alterations were found in many different regions of the brain, and the findings were conflicting; for example some studies showed increased whereas others showed decreased activation in the same regions. There is currently no conclusive hypothesis about what a decreased volume of certain brain regions means in terms of malfunction of a certain brain circuit. Moreover, when an activation (e.g. in terms of increased glucose metabolism) is observed in a particular brain centre, in comparisons to healthy controls, it is difficult to interpret what this activation means on a cellular or molecular basis. Does this mean that cells in this region are overactive or inactive because of a dysfunction of neurotransmitters or because of cell damage or does it instead reflect a dysfunction of the pathways passing through this region of interest? When blood flow is increased in a region of interest, does this mean that this special region is overactive, or another region behind this part of the brain? Moreover, several sources of artefacts may affect the interpretation of results. Another problem of brain imaging is the control of statistical errors—when there are many possibilities to compare certain brain regions with control samples, the probability increases that differences are found simply because of chance, and not due to real differences. Brain imaging studies may not yet be at a stage of delivering reliable results that could help to deepen understanding of the underlying mechanisms of pathological anxiety. At present, no therapeutic consequences can be derived from the available findings. However, it can be assumed that in the near future, brain imaging methods will play a crucial role in identifying brain systems that are altered in patients with anxiety disorders. The findings of brain imaging studies are summarized in reviews by Engel et al (2009) and Dresler et al (2013).

Early in the 1990s, brain imaging studies were performed with computed tomography (CT). In a number of CT studies, some distinct structural alterations in panic disorder patients were detected in small sample sizes. Most results were rather non-specific (e.g. demonstrating enlarged ventricles in the prefrontal cortex). Because of the low resolution of CT images, this method was abandoned in favour of magnetic resonance imaging (MRI), a method with a higher resolution. However, the results with structural MRI studies revealed hardly more specific on conclusive results.

Some studies have used functional imaging to investigate metabolism in certain regions of the brain. By using F-fluorodeoxyglucose positron emission tomography ({18FDG}-PET) with voxel-based analysis, an activation in glucose metabolism was found in certain brain regions associated with the anxiety network, e.g. the amygdala, hippocampus, or the thalamus. Regional blood flow was measured with Tc^{99m}-hexamethylpropylene amine oxime single-photon emission computed tomography (HM-PAO-SPECT) and was found to be reduced in certain frontal regions and increased in others. According to a review of imaging studies, patients with panic disorder showed abnormalities in limbic structure, in frontal and temporal areas, in the basal ganglia, and the brain stem (Dresler et al, 2013).

2.3.4 **Receptor binding and spectroscopic studies**

In search for a presumed dysfunction of GABA-ergic neurotransmission in panic disorder, binding to benzodiazepine binding sites was investigated by using radioactively marked receptor ligands such as flumazenil and iomazenil. Binding at serotonin ($5-HT_{1A}$) and dopamine receptors has also been investigated by using spectroscopy. In summary, alterations of GABA-ergic neurotransmission were found in frontal and temporal areas receptor binding studies in panic patients. In addition differences in serotonergic transmission, mainly in the raphe nuclei, were found (Dresler et al, 2013; Nikolaus et al, 2010).

2.3.5 **Provocation studies**

In some imaging studies, fear provocation techniques were used. The stimuli were potentially threatening words, words with negative emotional valence, anxiety related pictures, or pictures of faces with emotional expressions. However, the findings were inconsistent, some investigations finding activations, others finding decreased activity in the same regions. In some studies, panic attacks were provoked with lactate infusion, showing changes in regional blood flow in certain regions. However, the results of these studies are not easy to interpret, because sodium lactate may induce vasoconstriction. Also the drug yohimbine, used as another panic-provoking agent, causes vasoconstriction.

In a summary of provocations studies, the most consistent differences between panic patients and healthy controls were found in cingular, insular, frontal, and brain stem areas (Dresler et al, 2013).

2.3.6 **Neurochemistry**

Panic disorder has been associated with numerous claims of dysfunctions of neurotransmitter systems. Some hypotheses of neurobiological dysfunctions have been proposed involving the classical neurotransmitter systems such as serotonin, norepinephrine, and GABA.

2.3.6.1 *Serotonin*

Many drugs that enhance serotonergic neurotransmission, including SSRIs, serotonin-norepinephrine reuptake inhibitors (SNRIs), tricyclic antidepressants (TCAs), monoamine oxidase inhibitors (MAOIs), azapirones, and serotonin receptor antagonists, are effective in treating anxiety disorders. Therefore, it was assumed that a deficiency of the serotonin system may be a cause of pathological anxiety, and that serotonergic drugs exert their anxiolytic properties through inhibiting hyperexcited cells in brain regions belonging to the anxiety network by stimulation of serotonergic neurons.

Serotonergic neurons project from the raphe nuclei in the brainstem to regions in the brain that from the anxiety network, e.g. the amygdala, the hippocampus, the peri-aqueductal grey, the locus coeruleus, the hypothalamus, and the prefrontal cortex. Acute stress may increase serotonin turnover in these regions (Kent et al, 2002). However, rival theories exist with regard to a possible 5-HT deficiency versus excess: serotonin release may have both anxiogenic and anxiolytic effects, depending on the region of the forebrain involved. Also, the receptor type may play a role: anxiogenic effects are mediated by means of the $5-HT_{2A}$ receptor, whereas stimulation of $5-HT_{1A}$ receptors is anxiolytic. $5-HT_{1A}$ knockout mice show increased anxiety-like behaviours (Heisler et al, 1998).

Moreover, in patients with panic disorder, many possible dysfunctions of the serotonergic system have been investigated. Studies including measures of 5-HT in plasma, cerebrospinal fluid and platelets, challenge paradigms, and tryptophan depletion together show that the relationship between 5-HT and anxiety is complex (Bell and Nutt, 1998). Brain-imaging studies in panic patients demonstrate functional and clinically relevant alterations in various elements of 5-HT system affecting the neurocircuitry of panic. Genetic association studies suggest that certain 5-HT-related genes may contribute to a susceptibility to panic disorder; however, these data are limited and inconsistent. It appears that, even if not the primary aetiological factor in panic disorder, 5-HT function conveys important vulnerability as well as adaptive factors (Graeff, 2012; Maron and Shlik, 2006).

2.3.6.2 Norepinephrine

Medications that suppress both serotonin and norepinephrine reuptake, such as TCAs and SNRIs, are effective in treating anxiety disorders. It was assumed that the anxiolytic effects of these drugs were only due to their serotonergic component, because antidepressants with a predominantly noradrenergic component were less effective in panic disorder. However, the role of norepinephrine is uncertain, as reboxetine, a drug acting only as a norepinephrine reuptake inhibitor, was also effective in panic disorder.

The locus coeruleus, a small nucleus in the brain stem, contains 70% of all noradrenergic neurons in the brain. As the locus coeruleus plays an important role in anxiety mechanisms, it is assumed that noradrenergic mechanisms are central to this function. Stress activates the locus coeruleus, which results in increased norepinephrine release in projection sites of the locus coeruleus, including the amygdala, the prefrontal cortex, and the hippocampus. The locus coeruleus is activated by a variety of stressors (e.g. decreased blood volume or blood pressure), but also by external stress or threat. Activation of the locus coeruleus also stimulates the sympathetic nervous system and the HPA axis (Charney, 2004).

It assumed that in the prefrontal cortex, fear is perceived on a higher cognitive level, whereas the locus coeruleus is involved in instinctive fears. Activation of the locus coeruleus-norepinephrine system inhibits function of the prefrontal cortex, thereby favouring instinctual responses over more complex cognition (Charney and Bremner, 1999). Characteristically, in patients with panic disorder, rational considerations about the nature of anxiety are overridden by the 'primitive' anxiety system, and the locus coeruleus may be involved when the instinctive anxiety system takes control over intellectual reflections.

2.3.6.3 GABA

During stress and anxiety, GABA is released. By increasing chloride ion influx into the cell, GABA inhibits excited neurons. Benzodiazepines bind to the GABA receptor-complex and exert their anxiolytic effects by assisting GABA in decreasing hyperarousal in brain systems involved in anxiety. It was assumed that a so-called 'natural Valium' exists, i.e. an endogenous benzodiazepine ligand that is released in stress or fear situations. However, the existence of this ligand remains controversial.

Benzodiazepines are fast-acting anxiolytics. Some patients with panic disorder develop dependency on these drugs. The anxiolytic action of alcohol is also thought to be due to its action on GABA receptors. Alcohol is often abused by patients with anxiety disorders. Therefore, it was assumed that anxiety disorders may have their origin in a dysfunctional GABA-benzodiazepine receptor complex (Nutt and Malizia, 2001). In animals, exposure to inescapable stressors produces decreases in benzodiazepine receptor binding in the cortex. In patients with panic disorder, reduced benzodiazepine receptor binding has been found. These findings could be interpreted as a down-regulation of benzodiazepine receptor binding after exposure to stress. Other possible explanations are that stress results in changes in receptor affinity or changes in an endogenous ligand; or that a pre-existing low level of benzodiazepine receptor density may be a genetic risk factor for developing anxiety disorders.

2.3.6.4 CCK

CCK is a central nervous system neuropeptide involved in anxiety mechanisms, which is found in the cerebral cortex, the amygdala, the hippocampus, and other parts of the anxiety network. It antagonizes benzodiazepine effects (Bradwejn and de Montigny, 1984). Different forms exist (e.g. CCK-4 and CCK-8). CCK-4 given intravenously induces short panic-like states, and this effect is more marked in panic disorder patients than in healthy controls. Therefore, the substance is often used in panic-provocation studies in volunteers in order to study the neurobiology of anxiety. CCK-8S is increased in the cerebrospinal fluid of panic patients. A CCK-B antagonist was shown to block CCK-4-induced panic. Therefore, CCK antagonists were developed for the treatment of panic disorder, but these efforts were unsuccessful so far.

2.3.6.5 Neurokinins

Central neurokinins (tachykinins) have been shown to play a role in the modulation of stress-related behaviours and anxiety. Different forms exist: neurokinins (NK) 1, 2, and 3. Substance P, a ligand of the NK_1 receptor, has been found within brain areas known to be involved in the regulation of stress and anxiety responses (Ebner and Singewald, 2006). Neurokinin antagonists have been developed for the potential treatment of patients with anxiety disorders. Saredutant, a tachykinin NK_2 receptor antagonist, displayed mixed anxiolytic- and antidepressant-like activities in rodents. The drug has shown efficacy in major depression, but osanetant, NK_3-receptor antagonist, was not found effective in panic disorder (Kronenberg et al, 2005).

2.3.6.6 False suffocation alarm hypothesis

The influential 'suffocation false alarm' theory proposed by Klein (Klein, 1993) is a model assuming carbon-dioxide hypersensitivity in patients with panic disorder. The hypothesis postulates the existence of an evolved physiologic suffocation alarm system that monitors information about potential suffocation. Panic attacks maladaptively occur when the alarm is erroneously triggered. In this model, it is assumed that panic attacks are distinct from Cannon's emergency fear response and Selye's General Alarm Syndrome (Preter and Klein, 2008).

2.3.6.7 HPA function in psychiatric disorders

A dysfunctional hypothalamo-pituitary-adrenocortical (HPA) axis as the basis or a phenomenon in individuals with panic-disorder is an extensively investigated and discussed model. In response to stress, corticotropin-releasing hormone (CRH) is released from the hypothalamus into the hypothalamo-hypophyseal portal system. The portal system carries CRH to the pituitary, where it stimulates the release of corticotropin (adrenocorticotropin hormone, ACTH). Corticotropin stimulates the cortex of the adrenal gland and increases the synthesis of cortisol. Cortisol increases vigilance and mobilizes and replenishes energy stores. Increased cortisol levels have been found in normal individuals under stress provocation.

Numerous dysfunctions of the HPA axis have been found in patients with panic disorder, but these findings are inconsistent (Abelson et al, 2007). Baseline or basal state activity within the HPA axis is sometimes reported as elevated and sometimes as normal in patients with panic disorder. In 24-hour studies with frequent sampling, patients with panic disorder had normal daytime cortisol levels but some elevation overnight. Pharmacological probes like the dexamethasone suppression test have not demonstrated clear hypersuppression. CRH challenge has revealed blunted ACTH responses. Some 'panicogenic' stimuli (e.g. caffeine, sodium lactate, CO_2) can acutely trigger panic without a concomitant increase in cortisol release, while cortisol release by some of these laboratory panicogens has occasionally been reported. Spontaneous or natural panic attacks can occur without HPA axis activation. However, during unprovoked panic attacks in the patients' natural environment, a moderate cortisol increase was found (Bandelow et al, 2000).

At present it is not clear whether the dysfunctions of the HPA axis found in panic disorder are a potential cause of panic disorder, or just a consequence of permanent stress induced by recurrent panic attacks.

2.3.6.8 *Neuropeptide Y*

Neuropeptide Y is densely concentrated in brain regions involved in anxiety circuits, and has anxiolytic properties. It may also be involved in the consolidation of fear memories. Injection of neuropeptide Y into the amygdala reduces anxious behaviours and impairs memory retention of aversive stimuli. Neuropeptide Y reduces the firing of neurons in the locus coeruleus (Charney, 2004). Transgenic rats with neuropeptide Y over-expression have attenuated sensitivity to stress (Thorsell et al, 2000).

2.3.6.9 *The endogenous opioid system and the reward system*

The reward system, consisting of dopaminergic pathways from the ventral tegmental area to the nucleus accumbens, mediates responses to natural reinforcers, such as sex or food intake. The firing patterns of dopamine neurons are not only influenced by the reward itself, but also by the predictability of reward, i.e., they fire when rewards occur without being predicted or are better than predicted (Charney, 2004). The reward system also controls stress situations. When a punishment is predicted but does not take place, this is also followed by a release in the reward system. When we are in danger and expect to be hurt or killed but come out of this situation alive we are rewarded by a release of dopamine (perhaps explaining the ensuing 'high'). However, panic attacks are not followed by a release in the reward system. Although a patient experiencing a panic attack expects a 'punishment' (e.g. a myocardial infarction), the anticipated negative consequences do not occur. This unexpected escape from danger should be ensued by a release of the reward system. However, panic patients do not report euphoric feelings after an attack, but are usually left feeling depleted and exhausted.

The endogenous opioid system is directly connected with the brain reward system. Endorphins, the natural ligands of the opioid receptors, are released in stress situations. For example, an animal bleeding from many wounds from a fight with another, stronger animal, gets a release of endorphins, resulting in reduced pain and feelings of euphoria in order to be able to continue fighting for life. However, endorphins are also associated with many positive feelings, such as eating, hearing music, or winning in a lottery. The endogenous opioid system is also activated by positive social interactions, ranging from mutual grooming to sexual gratification. Opioid release results in feelings of comfort and alleviation of emotional distress arising from loss and social isolation (Panksepp, 2003).

Patients with panic disorder report a higher than normal rate of childhood separation anxiety and have a higher rate of actual childhood separation experiences (while these phenomena are not interrelated). Later in life, exacerbations of panic disorder may be associated with separation experiences (e.g. impending divorce). Therefore, a dysfunction of the opioid system in panic disorder has been hypothesized (Preter and Klein, 2008). Endogenous opioids protect healthy subjects from panic attacks, while endorphins increases suffocation sensitivity and separation anxiety in panic patients, making them more vulnerable to panic attacks (Graeff, 2012). This theory could at least explain panic attacks in patients with borderline personality disorder (BPD), which are quite common in this population. According to a recent theory, the neurobiology of BPD is based on a deficiency of the endogenous opiate system (EOS) (Bandelow et al, 2010b).

2.4 **Gender influences**

Like other anxiety disorders, panic disorder is more frequent in women in representative surveys. Several possible reasons for this phenomenon have been proposed and are listed in Box 2.1.

Box 2.1 Possible reasons for increased frequency of panic disorder in women

- *Psychosocial reasons*: In a world still largely dominated by men, women may have more reasons to be anxious. However, anxiety disorders mostly are characterised by unrealistic fears of harmless objects or situations, such as the fear of lifts, mice, or shopping malls, not by fears that represent a real threat (e.g. losing a job or being assaulted).
- *Difference in the expression of fears*: It was hypothesized that men, corresponding to their social role, hide their fears, while women express them more often, which results in higher reporting rates of anxiety disorders in women. However, then it could be expected that cultural influences also determine the higher rate in women, but there are no major differences between different cultures regarding the female-to-male ratio.
- *Female hormones*: Some data suggest that female reproductive hormones and related cycles may play an important role (Pigott, 1999). In animal models, female rats consistently show greater increases in corticosterone and ACTH in response to acute and chronic stressors. These differences have generally been attributed to the activational effects of gonadal steroids on elements of the HPA axis in females (Young et al, 2001). Several studies suggest that estradiol may play a role in enhanced stress responses in female rats. During pregnancy, panic symptoms are usually decreased in patients with panic disorder, while soon after childbirth, exacerbations of panic disorder have been reported (Bandelow et al, 2006). It is assumed that the sudden decreases in female hormones after delivery is the reason for this phenomenon.
- *Genetic reasons*: It was hypothesised that a greater anxiety vulnerability is genetically determined. Some genetic studies have found gender differences (Bandelow et al, 2010a; Domschke et al, 2004).

2.5 **Panic disorder and epilepsy**

In several investigations, EEG abnormalities were found in patients with panic disorder. Patients with epilepsy often develop panic attacks, and some patients have auras that resemble panic attacks. The amygdala/hippocampus region is a part of the brain which is most likely to be the focus of an epileptic fit. Therefore, it was assumed that a panic attack is has some similarities to an epileptiform seizure (Alvarez-Silva et al, 2006). Anticonvulsants have been used with success in small studies in patients with panic disorder. However, it is most likely that this theory applies only to a minority of panic patients.

2.6 **Summary: aetiology of panic disorder**

In this section, an aetiological model of panic disorder is summarized, by integrating findings from the various explanation models. In a perhaps over-simplified hypothetical model, pathological anxiety could be explained by a three-instance model, which somehow resembles Freud's structural model of the 'Id', the 'Super-Ego', and the 'Ego'. Translating the old psychoanalytic terms into new neurobiological language, the 'Id' would correspond to the brain reward system. The main purpose of this system is a striving to bring about the satisfaction of the instinctual needs (basic drives such as food and sex, i.e. to promote food intake and mating), in order to guarantee survival of the individual and of the species.

This system is antagonized by the anxiety network described above. This network partly corresponds to the Super-Ego, because it stands in opposition to the desires of the reward system and warns living beings of all kinds of dangers that might occur when they try to satisfy the needs of their reward system (e.g. of other animals that compete for the same prey or want to defend their preserve). Without this anxiety network, social life among humans would be impossible, because the reward system would pursue its goals unhindered, and we would break all social rules on our way to achieve our needs for sex and food. The responses of the reward system and the anxiety network are instinctual, follow relatively primitive rules and are partly unconscious.

A third system, more or less corresponding to Freud's 'Ego', involves higher cognitive functions. In this part of the brain, which is probably located in the prefrontal cortex, feelings of anxiety and fear break through to our consciousness. This brain system is capable of complex intellectual reflections about fears: e.g. 'my boss would be offended if I criticize him in public' or 'symptoms like irregular heartbeat, dyspnoea, and chest pain could be signs of a myocardial infarction'. It is also capable of reasonable considerations, such as: 'If my ECG and my lab tests are OK, there is no reason to assume that I have coronary heart disease'. Although this system has the highest intellectual capabilities, it is the weakest of all three systems. The reward system and the anxiety network have to guarantee our survival, therefore, they can override the prefrontal cortex in extreme situations.

In a healthy human being, these three systems work together, more or less in balance. In pathological anxiety, however, the anxiety network takes control over the prefrontal cortex. As a part of a survival safeguard, the anxiety network dominates the intellectual brain. In patients with panic disorder, exaggerated fear of having a severe medical illness overrules reasonable thinking. While the 'intelligent brain' argues that several ECGs and other medical examinations have been normal, the keyed-up anxiety network insists that something must be terribly wrong with the heart. This explains why many panic patients find it hard to be convinced that they are not medically ill. A disturbance in brain systems that have to monitor whether the body is threatened by real physical danger seems to cause an overreaction to harmless stimuli. It is the mismatch between not being in a fight or flight situation and the extreme symptoms that patients experience, which makes them assume that they are in real danger. Therefore, the patients seek an explanation for this phenomenon, and as a seemingly logical consequence, develop hypochondriacal fears. The intelligent brain develops theories of underlying severe medical conditions and therefore emphasises the need for medical examinations and treatments.

After some spontaneous attacks, patients develop agoraphobia, which is characterised by the tendency to avoid situations in which help by a physician might be unavailable.

The reasons for this hyperarousal of the anxiety system are yet unclear, but seem to be multifactorial. Panic disorder has a strong genetic component with an interaction of multiple risk genes, each with only a minor individual influence. Environmental factors contributing to the aetiology of the anxiety disorder include early traumatic experiences, such as long separation from parents or sexual abuse, but also stressful life events in later life, while the influence of child rearing styles seems to be very limited. Some lines of evidence point to long-lasting effects on neurobiological systems such as the HPA axis or GABA receptors, which might explain the influences of early trauma.

Several neurobiological differences have been found between patients with panic disorder and healthy individuals. Although panic disorder has usually developed by the age of 30 years, an inborn vulnerability may exist since birth. One of the most favoured neurobiological theories of panic disorder assumes a dysfunction of the serotonin system, as most drugs that enhance serotonergic neurotransmission are effective in panic disorder. Also, dysfunctions of other neurotransmitter systems (or a complex interaction of multiple systems) may be involved in the aetiology of panic disorder.

Finally higher rate of panic disorder in women is probably due to hormonal and/or genetic influences.

References and further reading

Abelson JL, Khan S, Liberzon I, Young EA (2007). HPA axis activity in patients with panic disorder: review and synthesis of four studies. *Depress Anxiety* **24**: 66–76.

Alsene K, Deckert J, Sand P, de Wit H (2003). Association between A2a receptor gene polymorphisms and caffeine-induced anxiety. *Neuropsychopharmacology* **28**: 1694–702.

Alvarez-Silva S, Alvarez-Rodriguez J, Perez-Echeverria MJ, Alvarez-Silva I (2006). Panic and epilepsy. *J Anxiety Disord* **20**: 353–62.

Bandelow B, Wedekind D, Pauls J, Broocks A, Hajak G, Rüther E (2000). Salivary cortisol in panic attacks. *American Journal of Psychiatry* **157**: 454–6.

Bandelow B, Álvarez Tichauer G, Späth C, Broocks A, Hajak G, Bleich S, Rüther E (2001). Separation anxiety and actual separation experiences during childhood in patients with panic disorder. *Can J Psychiatry* **46**: 948–52.

Bandelow B, Spath C, Tichauer GA, Broocks A, Hajak G, Ruther E (2002). Early traumatic life events, parental attitudes, family history, and birth risk factors in patients with panic disorder. *Compr Psychiatry* **43**: 269–78.

Bandelow B, Sojka F, Broocks A, Hajak G, Bleich S, Rüther E (2006). Panic disorder during pregnancy and postpartum period. *Eur Psychiatry* **21**: 495–500.

Bandelow B, Saleh K, Pauls J, Domschke K, Wedekind D, Falkai P (2010a). Insertion/deletion polymorphism in the gene for angiotensin converting enzyme (ACE) in panic disorder: A gender-specific effect? *World J Biol Psychiatry* **11**: 66–70.

Bandelow B, Schmahl C, Falkai P, Wedekind D (2010b). Borderline personality disorder: A dysregulation of the endogenous opioid system? *Psychol Rev* **117**: 623–36.

Bell CJ, Nutt DJ (1998). Serotonin and panic. *Br J Psychiatry* **172**: 465–71.

Bradwejn J, de Montigny C (1984). Benzodiazepines antagonize cholecystokinin-induced activation of rat hippocampal neurones. *Nature* **312**: 363–4.

Busch FN, Milrod BL, Singer MB (1999). Theory and technique in psychodynamic treatment of panic disorder. *J Psychother Pract Res* **8**: 234–42.

Charney D, Bremner D (1999). The neurobiology of anxiety disorders. In: Charney D, ed. *Neurobiology of Mental Illness*. Oxford: Oxford University Press, pp 494–517.

Charney DS (2004). Psychobiological mechanisms of resilience and vulnerability: implications for successful adaptation to extreme stress. *Am J Psychiatry* **161**: 195–216.

Crowe RR, Goedken R, Samuelson S, Wilson R, Nelson J, Noyes R, Jr. (2001). Genomewide survey of panic disorder. *Am J Med Genet* **105**: 105–9.

Deckert J, Nothen MM, Franke P, et al. (1998). Systematic mutation screening and association study of the A1 and A2a adenosine receptor genes in panic disorder suggest a contribution of the A2a gene to the development of disease. *Mol-Psychiatry* **3**: 81–5.

Deckert J, Catalano M, Syagailo YV, et al. (1999). Excess of high activity monoamine oxidase A gene promoter alleles in female patients with panic disorder. *Hum-Mol-Genet* **8**: 621–4.

Domschke K, Dannlowski U (2010). Imaging genetics of anxiety disorders. *Neuroimage* **53**: 822–31.

Domschke K, Deckert J (2012) Genetics of anxiety disorders – status quo and quo vadis, *Curr Pharm Des* **18**: 5691–8

Domschke K, Freitag CM, Kuhlenbaumer G, et al. (2004). Association of the functional V158M catechol-O-methyl-transferase polymorphism with panic disorder in women. *Int J Neuropsychopharmacol* **7**: 183–8.

Domschke K, Braun M, Ohrmann P, et al. (2006). Association of the functional -1019C/G 5-HT1A polymorphism with prefrontal cortex and amygdala activation measured with 3 T fMRI in panic disorder. *Int J Neuropsychopharmacol* **9**: 349–55.

Domschke K, Deckert J, O'Donovan M C, Glatt SJ (2007). Meta-analysis of COMT val158met in panic disorder: ethnic heterogeneity and gender specificity. *Am J Med Genet B Neuropsychiatr Genet* **144**: 667–73.

Domschke K, Ohrmann P, Braun M, et al. (2008). Influence of the catechol-O-methyltransferase val158met genotype on amygdala and prefrontal cortex emotional processing in panic disorder. *Psychiatry Res* **163**: 13–20.

Domschke K, Reif A, Weber H, et al. (2011). Neuropeptide S receptor gene -- converging evidence for a role in panic disorder. *Mol Psychiatry* **16**: 938–48.

Domschke K, Tidow N, Kuithan H, et al. (2012). Monoamine oxidase A gene DNA hypomethylation - a risk factor for panic disorder? *Int J Neuropsychopharmacol* **15**: 1217–28.

Dresler T, Guhn A, Tupak SV, et al. (2013). Revise the revised? New dimensions of the neuroanatomical hypothesis of panic disorder. *J Neural Transm* **120**: 3–29.

Ebner K, Singewald N (2006). The role of substance P in stress and anxiety responses. *Amino Acids* **31**: 251–72.

Engel K, Bandelow B, Gruber O, Wedekind D (2009). Neuroimaging in anxiety disorders. *J Neural Transm* **116**: 703–16.

Erhardt A, Czibere L, Roeske D, et al. (2011). TMEM132D, a new candidate for anxiety phenotypes: evidence from human and mouse studies. *Mol Psychiatry* **16**: 647–63.

Faravelli C, Webb T, Ambonetti A, Fonnesu F, Sessarego A (1985). Prevalence of traumatic early life events in 31 agoraphobic patients with panic attacks. *Am J Psychiatry* **142**: 1493–4.

Freud S (1964). *Ueber die Berechtigung, von der Neurasthenie einen bestimmten Symptomencomplex als 'Angstneurose' abzutrennen (S. 319). Gesammelte Werke I.* (1895). Fischer, Frankfurt

Fuchs E, Flügge G (2006). Experimental animal models for the simulation of depression and anxiety. *Dialogues Clin Neurosci* **8**: 323–33.

Fyer AJ, Hamilton SP, Durner M, et al. (2006). A third-pass genome scan in panic disorder: evidence for multiple susceptibility loci. *Biol Psychiatry* **60**: 388–401.

Gelernter J, Bonvicini K, Page G, et al. (2001). Linkage genome scan for loci predisposing to panic disorder or agoraphobia. *Am J Med Genet* **105**: 548–57.

Gorman JM, Kent JM, Sullivan GM, Coplan JD (2000). Neuroanatomical hypothesis of panic disorder, revised. *American Journal of Psychiatry* **157**: 493–505.

Graeff FG (2012). New perspective on the pathophysiology of panic: merging serotonin and opioids in the periaqueductal gray. *Braz J Med Biol Res* **45**: 366–75.

Hamilton SP, Slager SL, Heiman GA, et al. (2002). Evidence for a susceptibility locus for panic disorder near the catechol-O-methyltransferase gene on chromosome 22. *Biol Psychiatry* **51**: 591–601.

Hamilton SP, Slager SL, De Leon AB, et al. (2004). Evidence for genetic linkage between a polymorphism in the adenosine 2A receptor and panic disorder. *Neuropsychopharmacology* **29**: 558–65.

Heisler LK, Chu HM, Brennan TJ, Danao JA, Bajwa P, Parsons LH, Tecott LH (1998). Elevated anxiety and antidepressant-like responses in serotonin 5-HT1A receptor mutant mice. *Proc Natl Acad Sci U S A* **95**: 15049–54.

Hettema JM, Neale MC, Kendler KS (2001). A review and meta-analysis of the genetic epidemiology of anxiety disorders. *Am J Psychiatry* **158**: 1568–78.

Hosing VG, Schirmacher A, Kuhlenbaumer G, et al. (2004). Cholecystokinin- and cholecystokinin-B-receptor gene polymorphisms in panic disorder. *J Neural Transm Suppl* 147–56.

Kaabi B, Gelernter J, Woods SW, Goddard A, Page GP, Elston RC (2006). Genome scan for loci predisposing to anxiety disorders using a novel multivariate approach: strong evidence for a chromosome 4 risk locus. *Am J Hum Genet* **78**: 543–53.

Kennedy JL, Bradwejn J, Koszycki D, King N, Crowe R, Vincent J, Fourie O (1999). Investigation of cholecystokinin system genes in panic disorder. *Mol-Psychiatry* **4**: 284–5.

Kent JM, Mathew SJ, Gorman JM (2002). Molecular targets in the treatment of anxiety. *Biol Psychiatry* **52**: 1008–30.

Kessler RC, Berglund P, Demler O, Jin R, Merikangas KR, Walters EE (2005). Lifetime prevalence and age-of-onset distributions of DSM-IV disorders in the National Comorbidity Survey Replication. *Arch Gen Psychiatry* **62**: 593–602.

Klauke B, Deckert J, Reif A, et al. (2011). Serotonin transporter gene and childhood trauma—a G x E effect on anxiety sensitivity. *Depress Anxiety* **28**: 1048–57.

Klauke B, Deckert J, Zwanzger P, et al. (2012). Neuropeptide S receptor gene (NPSR) and life events: G x E effects on anxiety sensitivity and its subdimensions. *World J Biol Psychiatry*

Klein DF (1993). False suffocation alarms, spontaneous panics, and related conditions. An integrative hypothesis. *Archives of General Psychiatry* **50**: 306–17.

Knowles JA, Fyer AJ, Vieland VJ, et al. (1998). Results of a genome-wide genetic screen for panic disorder. *Am-J-Med-Genet* **81**: 139–47.

Kronenberg G, Berger P, Tauber RF, Bandelow B, Henkel V, Heuser I (2005). Randomized, double blind study of SR142801 (onasetant). A novel neurokinin-3 (NK3) receptor antagonist in panic disorder with pre- and posttreatment cholecystokinin tetrapeptide (CCK-4) challenges. *Pharmacopsychiatry* **38**: 24–29.

LeDoux JE, Cicchetti P, Xagoraris A, Romanski LM (1990). The lateral amygdaloid nucleus: sensory interface of the amygdala in fear conditioning. *J Neurosci* **10**: 1062–9.

LeDoux JE (1996). *The Emotional Brain: The Mysterious Underpinnings of Emotional Life*. Simon & Schuster, New York

Lonsdorf TB, Ruck C, Bergstrom J, Andersson G, Ohman A, Lindefors N, Schalling M (2010). The COMTval158met polymorphism is associated with symptom relief during exposure-based cognitive-behavioral treatment in panic disorder. *BMC Psychiatry* **10**: 99.

Maier W, Lichtermann D, Minges J, Oehrlein A, Franke P (1993). A controlled family study in panic disorder. *J Psychiatr Res* **27**(Suppl 1): 79–87.

Maron E, Shlik J (2006). Serotonin function in panic disorder: important, but why? *Neuropsychopharmacology* **31**: 1–11.

Mellman TA, Uhde TW (1990). Patients with frequent sleep panic: clinical findings and response to medication treatment. *J Clin Psychiatry* **51**: 513–6.

Nikolaus S, Antke C, Beu M, Muller HW (2010). Cortical GABA, striatal dopamine and midbrain serotonin as the key players in compulsive and anxiety disorders-results from in vivo imaging studies. *Rev Neurosci* **21**: 119–39.

Nocon A, Wittchen HU, Beesdo K, et al. (2008). Differential familial liability of panic disorder and agoraphobia. *Depress Anxiety* **25**: 422–34.

Nutt DJ, Malizia AL (2001). New insights into the role of the GABA(A)-benzodiazepine receptor in psychiatric disorder. *Br J Psychiatry* **179**: 390–6.

Panksepp J (2003). Neuroscience. Feeling the pain of social loss. *Science* **302**: 237–9.

Perna G, Favaron E, Di Bella D, Bussi R, Bellodi L (2005). Antipanic efficacy of paroxetine and polymorphism within the promoter of the serotonin transporter gene. *Neuropsychopharmacology* **30**: 2230–5.

Pigott TA (1999). Gender differences in the epidemiology and treatment of anxiety disorders. *J Clin Psychiatry* **60**: 4–15.

Preter M, Klein DF (2008). Panic, suffocation false alarms, separation anxiety and endogenous opioids. *Progress in Neuro-Psychopharmacology & Biological Psychiatry* **32**: 603–12.

Reif A, Weber H, Domschke K, et al. (2012). Meta-analysis argues for a female-specific role of MAOA-uVNTR in panic disorder in four European populations. *Am J Med Genet B Neuropsychiatr Genet* **159B**: 786–93. Epub Date 2013/01/16.

Reif A, Richter J, Straube B, et al. (2013). MAOA and mechanisms of panic disorder revisited: from bench to molecular psychotherapy. *Mol Psychiatry*

Rothe C, Koszycki D, Bradwejn J, et al. (2006). Association of the Val158Met catechol O-methyltransferase genetic polymorphism with panic disorder. *Neuropsychopharmacology* **31**: 2237–42.

Saeki Y, Watanabe T, Ueda M, et al. (2009). Genetic and pharmacokinetic factors affecting the initial pharmacotherapeutic effect of paroxetine in Japanese patients with panic disorder. *Eur J Clin Pharmacol* **65**: 685–91.

Samochowiec J, Hajduk A, Samochowiec A, Horodnicki J, Stepien G, Grzywacz A, Kucharska-Mazur J (2004). Association studies of MAO-A, COMT, and 5-HTT genes polymorphisms in patients with anxiety disorders of the phobic spectrum. *Psychiatry Res* **128**: 21–6.

Seligman MEP (1971). Phobias and preparedness. *Behavior Therapy* **2**: 307–320.

Stein MB, Schork NJ, Gelernter J (2008). Gene-by-environment (serotonin transporter and childhood maltreatment) interaction for anxiety sensitivity, an intermediate phenotype for anxiety disorders. *Neuropsychopharmacology* **33**: 312–9.

Thorgeirsson TE, Oskarsson H, Desnica N, et al. (2003). Anxiety with panic disorder linked to chromosome 9q in Iceland. *Am J Hum Genet* **72**: 1221–30.

Thorsell A, Michalkiewicz M, Dumont Y, et al. (2000). Behavioral insensitivity to restraint stress, absent fear suppression of behavior and impaired spatial learning in transgenic rats with hippocampal neuropeptide Y overexpression. *Proc Natl Acad Sci U S A* **97**: 12852–7.

Vieland VJ, Goodman DW, Chapman T, Fyer AJ (1996). New segregation analysis of panic disorder. *Am-J-Med-Genet* **67**: 147–53.

Yevtushenko OO, Oros MM, Reynolds GP (2010). Early response to selective serotonin reuptake inhibitors in panic disorder is associated with a functional 5-HT1A receptor gene polymorphism. *J Affect Disord* **123**: 308–11.

Young EA, Altemus M, Parkison V, Shastry S (2001). Effects of estrogen antagonists and agonists on the ACTH response to restraint stress in female rats. *Neuropsychopharmacology* **25**: 881–91.

Chapter 3

Pharmacological treatment

Key points

- First-line treatment should be with selective serotonin reuptake inhibitors (SSRIs) or serotonin norepinephrine reuptake inhibitors (SNRIs)
- The treatment effect of antidepressants emerges slowly, over 2–4 weeks
- Treatment should be continued for one year or more
- Second-line treatments include TCAs or MAOIs
- Benzodiazepines may be used in combination with antidepressants during the first weeks, before the onset of effect of the antidepressants; or in patients in whom other treatments were not effective or were not tolerated due to side effects

3.1 Introduction

Anxiety symptoms exist on a continuum and many people with milder degrees of anxiety will experience an improvement without specific intervention. Some patients have only very infrequent panic attacks and may not need treatment at all, if the clinical picture is not complicated by anticipatory anxiety or agoraphobia. However, all patients fulfilling the complete criteria of panic disorder should obtain treatment.

Drugs available for the treatment of panic disorder are listed in Table 3.1. These recommendations are based on randomized, double-blind clinical studies published in peer-reviewed journals. Over 200 controlled trials have been performed in patients with panic disorder. These treatment studies were evaluated by the World Federation of Societies of Biological Psychiatry Task Force on Treatment Guidelines for Anxiety, Obsessive–Compulsive and Post-Traumatic Stress Disorders, a panel of 30 international anxiety experts (Bandelow et al, 2008). To be recommended, a drug must have shown its efficacy in double-blind placebo-controlled (DBPC) studies. When an established standard treatment exists for a specific disorder, a drug must have been compared with this reference drug (comparator trial). The studies had to fulfil certain methodological standards. Due to space limits, the references of these studies are not given here. Not all of the recommended drugs are licensed for these indications in every country.

All drugs for panic disorder have advantages and disadvantages, summarized in Table 3.2.

Table 3.1 Recommendations for drug treatment of panic disorder*

Treatment	Examples	Recommended daily dose for adults (mg)
Treatment of acute panic attacks		
Benzodiazepines	Alprazolam, Lorazepam melting tablets	0.5–2 1–2.5
Standard treatment		
SSRIs	Citalopram	20–60
	Escitalopram	10–20
	Fluoxetine	20–40
	Fluvoxamine	100–300
	Paroxetine	20–60
	Sertraline	50–200
SNRI	Venlafaxine	75–225
TCA	Clomipramine	75–250
	Imipramine	75–250

*Not all drugs mentioned are currently approved in all countries for panic disorder, in the populations, or at the doses being discussed.

Table 3.2 Advantages and disadvantages of antianxiety drugs

Medication class	Advantages	Disadvantages	Side effects
Selective serotonin reuptake inhibitors (SSRIs)	No dependency Sufficient evidence from clinical studies Favourable side effect profile Relatively safe in overdose	Latency of effect 2–6 weeks	Initial jitteriness, nausea, restlessness, sexual dysfunction, and other side effects
Serotonin norepinephrine reuptake inhibitor— venlafaxine (SNRI)	No dependency Sufficient evidence from clinical studies Favourable side effect profile Relatively safe in overdose	Latency of effect 2–6 weeks	Initial jitteriness, nausea, restlessness, sexual dysfunction, increase of blood pressure in high doses and other side effects
Tricyclic antidepressants (TCA)	No dependency Sufficient evidence from clinical studies	Latency of effect 2–6 weeks	Anticholinergic effects, cardiovascular side effects, weight gain and other side effects, sexual dysfunction May be lethal in overdose

Table 3.2 Advantages and disadvantages of antianxiety drugs			
Medication class	Advantages	Disadvantages	Side effects
Irreversible monoamine-oxidase inhibitor phenelzine (MAOI)	No dependency	Latency of effect 2–6 weeks Food–drug interactions possible; dietary restrictions required Multiple daily dosing needed	Activation, insomnia, weight gain, orthostatic hypotension, sexual dysfunctions, gastrointestinal, and other side effects May be lethal in overdose
Benzodiazepines	Rapid onset of action Sufficient evidence from clinical studies Relatively safe in overdose		Dependency possible; sedation, slow reaction time, and other side effects

3.2 Selective serotonin reuptake inhibitors (SSRIs)

The efficacy of SSRIs in panic disorder has been established through many randomized placebo-controlled studies, and they are widely considered to be the first-line drugs for this disorder. Efficacy has been shown for all available SSRIs. Usually, treatment with SSRIs is well tolerated. Restlessness, jitteriness, an increase in anxiety symptoms, and insomnia in the first days or weeks of treatment may hamper compliance with treatment. Lowering the starting dose of SSRIs may make this less troublesome. Other side effects include fatigue, dizziness, nausea, loss of appetite, or weight gain. Sexual dysfunction (decreased libido, erectile dysfunction, or ejaculatory disturbance) may be a problem in long-term treatment, and discontinuation syndromes have been observed. The anxiolytic effect may start with a latency of 2–4 weeks (in some cases up to 6–8 weeks). To avoid overstimulation and insomnia, doses should be given in the morning and at midday, except in patients reporting daytime sedation.

SSRIs inhibit the reuptake of serotonin from the synaptic cleft to the presynaptic neuron. By increasing the amount of serotonin in the cleft, they enhance neurotransmission in serotonergic pathways. It is still speculative how SSRIs exhibit their anxiolytic properties: but serotonergic neurons project from the raphe nuclei in the brainstem to regions in the brain that form the anxiety network, and by inhibiting hyperexcited cells in these regions, SSRIs may dampen down exaggerated fear reactions.

3.3 Serotonin-norepinephrine reuptake inhibitors (SNRIs)

The efficacy of the antidepressant venlafaxine, a selective serotonin norepinephrine reuptake-inhibitor, was demonstrated in placebo-controlled studies and in comparisons with reference drugs. The side effect profile of venlafaxine is similar to the SSRIs. When using higher doses (300 mg/day or more), blood pressure should be monitored. SNRIs do not only enhance serotonergic transmission, but also block the reuptake of norepinephrine. It is still not clear whether the anxiolytic properties of the SNRIs are solely due to the serotonergic component or are also mediated through the dual reuptake inhibition.

3.4 Tricyclic antidepressants (TCAs)

Treatment with some TCAs (imipramine, clomipramine) has been shown to improve panic disorder. Especially at the beginning of treatment, compliance may be hampered by adverse effects such as initially increased anxiety, dry mouth, postural hypotension, tachycardia, sedation, sexual dysfunction, impaired psychomotor function, impaired driving, and other side effects. Weight gain may be a problem in long-term treatment. In general, the frequency of adverse events is higher for TCAs than for newer antidepressants, such as the SSRIs or SNRIs. TCAs should be avoided in patients considered at risk of suicide, due to their potential cardiac and central nervous system (CNS) toxicity after overdose. The dosage should be titrated up slowly until dosage levels as high as in the treatment of depression are reached. Patients should be informed that the onset of the anxiolytic effect of the drug may have a latency of 2–4 weeks (in some cases up to 6–8 weeks).

Tricyclic antidepressants inhibit both serotonin and norepinephrine reuptake. Additionally, they block other receptor systems, such as the cholinergic system, which is associated with side effects. Antihistaminergic properties are associated with sedation, which may be advantageous at the beginning of treatment, but can also lead to unwanted drowsiness in the long term.

3.5 Benzodiazepines

Benzodiazepines bind to the gamma-aminobutyric acid (GABA) receptor complex and exert their anxiolytic effects by assisting GABA in 'calming down' hyperarousal in brain systems involved in anxiety. The efficacy of benzodiazepines in panic disorder has been shown in controlled clinical studies with alprazolam, clonazepam, lorazepam, and diazepam.

The anxiolytic effects start almost immediately after oral or parenteral application. In contrast to antidepressants, benzodiazepines do not lead to initially increased nervousness. Due to CNS depression, benzodiazepine treatment may be associated with sedation, dizziness, prolonged reaction time and other side effects. Cognitive functions and driving skills may be affected. After long-term treatment with benzodiazepines (e.g. over 4–8 months), dependency may occur in some patients, especially in predisposed patients. Withdrawal reactions have their peak severity at 2 days for short half-life and 4–7 days for long half-life benzodiazepines. Tolerance seems to be rare, but it is claimed that prolonged withdrawal reactions may occasionally occur. Thus, treatment with benzodiazepines requires careful weighing of the potential risks and anticipated benefits. There is some controversy in the field as to whether benzodiazepines can be used as first-line agents in anxiety disorders. In patients in whom other treatment modalities were not effective or were not tolerated due to side effects, year-long treatment with benzodiazepines may be justified. However, patients with a history of benzodiazepine abuse should be excluded from treatment. Cognitive-behavioural interventions may facilitate benzodiazepine discontinuation. Benzodiazepines may also be used in combination with antidepressants during the first weeks before the onset of efficacy of the antidepressants. When treating patients with comorbid panic disorder, one should be aware that benzodiazepines, in contrast to antidepressants, do not treat comorbid conditions such as depression or obsessive–compulsive disorder.

3.6 Monoamine oxidase inhibitors (MAOI)

Despite the widespread use of phenelzine in panic disorder, evidence of efficacy is only based on one randomized controlled trial (RCT). In this study, phenelzine was superior to placebo and equal in efficacy to imipramine, or even superior on some measures. However, because of the possibility of severe side effects and interactions with other drugs or food components, the MAOI phenelzine is not considered a first-line drug and should only be used by experienced psychiatrists when other treatment modalities have been unsuccessful or have not been tolerated. To avoid overstimulation and insomnia, doses should be given in the morning and at midday.

MAOIs block the enzyme monoamine oxidase, leading to a decreased metabolization of serotonin to 5-hydroxy-indolacetic acid. Therefore, serotonergic neurotransmission is enhanced because more serotonin is available in the cell. Also, the metabolism of other neurotransmitters like norepinephrine and dopamine is blocked by MAOIs.

3.7 Other medications

Other medications that have been investigated in panic disorder are listed in Section 3.11. These may be considered as 'off-label' treatments for treatment-refractory patients. Some drugs have shown negative results in panic disorder. These include propranolol, buspirone, and bupropion.

3.8 Comparisons of antipanic drugs

In studies comparing the efficacy of TCAs and SSRIs, no differences in terms of efficacy could be found between the two classes of drugs, with the exception of maprotiline, which had no effect in contrast to fluvoxamine. However, in most of these studies, the SSRIs were better tolerated than the TCAs. Comparisons among the SSRIs did not reveal differences with regard to efficacy in general, although escitalopram shows evidence of superiority over citalopram on some outcome measures (Bandelow et al, 2007).

There are no direct comparisons between SSRIs and benzodiazepines in the treatment of panic disorder. According to a meta-analysis, effect sizes for the SSRIs were somewhat higher than for the benzodiazepine alprazolam.

In a number of studies, alprazolam was compared with the tricyclic antidepressant imipramine. No differences could be found between the two drugs in terms of global improvement.

The advantages and disadvantages of antipanic drugs are summarized in Table 3.2.

3.9 Long-term treatment

In most patients, panic disorder has a waxing and waning course. After remission, treatment should continue for at least several months in order to prevent relapse. A number of studies have investigated the long-term value of SSRI and TCA treatment. Some of these trials are long-term studies comparing a drug and placebo for a longer period (i.e. 26–60 weeks). The other type of trials are relapse prevention studies, in which patients usually receive open label treatment with the study drug for a shorter period, after which responders are randomized to receive ongoing active drug treatment or placebo. In summary, SSRIs, the SNRI venlafaxine, TCAs and moclobemide showed long-term efficacy in these studies.

Data on how long maintenance treatment should be continued are scarce. In one study, patients who had 18 months of maintenance treatment with imipramine had fewer relapses after discontinuation than did patients who were discontinued after only 6 months of treatment. The results support the hypothesis that successful imipramine maintenance treatment of patients with panic and agoraphobia can have protective effects against relapse, at least in the first 6 months after the maintenance treatment period.

Expert consensus conferences generally recommend continuing drug treatment for at least 12 months. Regarding SSRIs, the same doses are usually prescribed in the maintenance treatment of panic disorder as in the acute treatment phase. To our knowledge, there are no studies examining reduced doses of SSRIs in maintenance treatment. In an open study with the TCA imipramine, patients stabilized on imipramine received further treatment with half their previous dose of imipramine, did not show relapse or sustained worsening.

3.10 **Practical guidelines for treatment**

Recommended dosages are indicated in Table 3.1. SSRIs have a flat dose-response curve, i.e. approximately 75% of patients respond to the initial (low) dose. However, for paroxetine, a dosage of 40 mg/day has been found more effective than 20 mg/day.

In some patients, treatment may be started with half the recommended dose in the first days or weeks. Patients with panic disorder are sensitive to antidepressants and may easily discontinue treatment because of initial jitteriness and nervousness.

For TCAs, it is recommended to initiate the drug at a low dose and to increase dosage every 3–5 days. The antidepressant dose should be increased to the highest recommended level when initial treatment with a low or medium dosage is ineffective. In order to increase compliance, it may be feasible to give all the antidepressant medication in a single dose, depending upon the patient's tolerance. Benzodiazepine dosage should be as low as possible but as high as necessary to achieve a complete treatment result.

Panic disorder has a chronic course. Therefore some patients express the fear that they have to take medication for 'the rest of their life'. However, treatment over many years is more the exception than the rule. The anxiety disorder has a waxing and waning course. This can be demonstrated by the description of a typical case.

A patient with panic disorder starts treatment at the age of 36 and his psychiatrist recommends taking a drug for 1 year. Then, treatment is tapered off, and the patient does not require treatment for another 2 years. Then again, a period of panic attacks could occur, requiring another year of drug intake. This pattern may be repeated for another two or three periods. When getting older, the healthy intervals get longer, and the panic periods are attenuated. The patient learns to cope with his problem and to get along without drug treatment. By the age of 45, the panic attacks slowly become

Table 3.3 Treatment of panic disorder: frequently asked questions	
Question	Answer
How can compliance be improved?	Inform patient about the delayed onset of action and possible side effects, which might occur in the first weeks of treatment (such as insomnia or restlessness with SSRIs/SNRIs)
Can medication be stopped after onset of efficacy?	Expert conferences recommend extending treatment for at least 1 year to avoid relapses
Will drug treatment be life-long?	In most patients, symptoms of panic disorder usually lessen after the age of 45. The disorder has a waxing and waning course. Therefore, only a proportion of patients may require treatment lasting longer than a few years
Is there a possibility for irreversible side-effects after year-long treatment?	There is no evidence of irreversible side effects with SSRIs, SNRIs, or TCAs
Which doses are used in maintenance treatment?	SSRIs should be used the same dosages as in acute treatment, while TCAs may be used in half the dose recommended for acute treatment
When should treatment be stopped because of lack of efficacy?	After 4–6 weeks
What if partial response occurs after 4–6 weeks?	Treat for another 4–6 weeks with increased dose before changing the treatment strategy
Can antipanic drugs be combined?	Usually monotherapy is the better option. Combinations of drugs may be used in treatment-resistant cases. Benzodiazepines may be used in combination in the first weeks before onset of efficacy of the antidepressants
Should medication be stopped before starting cognitive behaviour therapy?	There is no evidence that drugs may weaken the effects of CBT; in contrast, meta-analyses have shown that combination of both treatment modalities is more effective than both monotherapies

less frequent and eventually disappear completely. In his whole life span, the patients had needed to take the antipanic medication 4 to 5 years.

Some 'Frequently Asked Questions' for the treatment of panic disorder are summarized in Table 3.3.

3.11 **Management of treatment-resistant panic disorder**

Many patients continue to experience recurrent panic attacks, agoraphobic avoidance, or continuing distress and impairment. According to clinical studies, around 20–40% of patients treated with standard treatments remain symptomatic. In naturalistic settings, this percentage may be even higher, as the patients selected in clinical studies are often less severely ill, younger, and have less comorbid conditions than the general patient population.

A number of risk factors predicting poorer outcome of treatment have been identified, including:

- long duration of illness
- high baseline illness severity
- severe agoraphobic avoidance
- strong hypochondriacal fears
- frequent emergency room visits
- comorbidity with other anxiety disorders, depression, or personality disorders
- reduced general mental health
- unemployment
- delayed response to medication
- low treatment compliance with a cognitive behaviour therapy regimen.

A 'treatment-resistant' patient could be defined as someone who had a standard treatment for a minimum of 6 weeks without showing response. The definition of treatment non-response or partial response may be somehow arbitrary. Psychiatric rating scales may provide an objective measure. Analogous to guidelines for the use of rating scales in new drug application, response could be defined as a 50% reduction on a standard rating scale, such as the Panic and Agoraphobia Scale (Bandelow, 1999) (see Appendix 2). Similarly, 'partial' response could be defined as a 25% reduction of scale scores.

When initial treatment fails, a decision needs to be made about when to change medication. Controlled data are lacking for panic disorder. If partial response is seen after 4–6 weeks, there is still a chance that the patient will respond after another 4–6 weeks of therapy with an increased dose. However, if the patient shows no evidence of any response to treatment at adequate dosage after 4–6 weeks, the medication should be changed.

Little data exist on dose escalations in patients who failed to obtain a satisfactory response with standard doses. In one study (Michelson et al, 2001), patients who had failed to achieve adequate response to 20 mg fluoxetine daily were successfully treated with increased doses of up to 60 mg fluoxetine daily.

Before a treatment is considered a failure, possible other reasons for non-responsiveness should be considered (Box 3.1).

It should be ascertained that the diagnosis is correct, the patient is compliant with therapy, the dosage prescribed is therapeutic, and there has been an adequate trial

Box 3.1 Check list for non-response
Is the diagnosis correct?
Is the patient compliant with treatment?
Adequate dosage?
Adequate treatment duration?
Interactions with other medication or food?
Fast metaboliser?
Comorbid psychiatric or medical conditions that may lead to poor outcome?

period. Concurrent prescription of other drugs may interfere with efficacy, such as metabolic enhancers or inhibitors. Some patients metabolize drugs very quickly. Although the determination of plasma levels is not used routinely due to the low correlations between oral dose and plasma levels or between plasma levels and clinical effect, this may help to identify patients who do not take their medication at all or are fast metabolizers. Psychosocial factors may affect response, and depression, borderline personality disorder, and substance abuse are especially likely to complicate panic disorder.

Treatment strategies for patients failing to respond to standard treatments are summarized in Table 3.4.

Table 3.4 Treatment options for patients failing to respond to initial standard treatments. Some of the suggestions have to be regarded as off-label treatment		
Strategy	Example	Evidence
Combining drug treatment and psychotherapy	Combination of SSRIs and CBT	Combination more effective than monotherapies
Switching to another first-line treatment	Switching from one SSRI to another	Effective in RCTs, but switching studies are lacking
	Switching from venlafaxine to an SSRI or vice versa	Effective in RCTs, but switching studies are lacking
Switching to second-line treatments	Switching to TCAs	Effective in RCTs, but switching studies are lacking
	Switching to benzodiazepines	Effective in RCTs, but switching studies are lacking
	Switching to phenelzine	Effective in RCTs, but switching studies are lacking
Combinations of first- and second-line drugs	Combining SSRIs and benzodiazepines	According to a DBPC study, combined treatment resulted in more rapid response than with the SSRI alone, but there was no differential benefit beyond the initial few weeks of therapy
	Combining SSRIs with TCAs	No published studies
Switching to drugs that were effective in other anxiety disorders	Pregabalin	Effective in a number of RCTs in generalized anxiety disorder
	Duloxetine	Effective in a number of RCTs in generalized anxiety disorder
	Quetiapine	Effective in a number of RCTs in generalized anxiety disorder
	Agomelatine	Effective in a number of RCTs in generalized anxiety disorder

(continued)

Table 3.4 (continued)		
Switching to treatments with preliminary evidence	Mirtazapine	As effective as fluvoxamine in an RCT (study inconclusive due to lack of power)
	Inositol	Superior to placebo and as effective as in RCTs
Switching to treatments with inconsistent results	Reboxetine	Effective in a DBPC study. In a single-blind study the drug was equally effective as fluvoxamine (Seedat et al., 2003), but less effective than paroxetine. Not available in many countries
	Moclobemide	Inconsistent results in RCTs
	Gabapentin	Only superior to placebo in more severely ill panic patients
	Tiagabine	Effective in a case series, but inconsistent results in generalized anxiety disorder
Switching to treatments only tested in cases series	Vigabatrin	Effective in a small case series
	Milnacipran	Effective in a small case series
Treatments studied in treatment-resistant cases	Pindolol augmentation	Effective in a DBPC study
	Switch from citalopram to reboxetine and vice versa	Effective in a single-blind study
	Adding of fluoxetine to a TCA or vice versa	Effective in a small open study
	Valproate + clonazepam	Effective in a case series
	Clomipramine + lithium	Effective in one case report
	Olanzapine	Effective in a case series
	Addition of olanzapine to ongoing treatment	Effective in case reports
	Adding CBT in patients unresponsive to drug treatment	Effective in studies without control condition for CBT
	Adding SSRIs or clomipramine to patients unresponsive to CBT	Effective in DBPC studies

CBT, cognitive behavioural therapy; DBPC, double blind placebo-controlled; RCT, randomized controlled trial.

Few studies are available to guide selection of treatment for patients with treatment-resistant panic disorder. Data from controlled clinical studies with regular panic patients are not easily transferable to treatment-resistant cases.

As a first measure, it seems rational to switch from one standard treatment to another. Although 'switching studies' are lacking, the current clinical consensus is that a patient who has failed a single trial of an SSRI should be switched to another SSRI or to the SNRI venlafaxine. The next step would be to change to a TCA. Then, benzodiazepines should be tried. Although the data with the reversible inhibitor of monoamine-oxidase A moclobemide were inconsistent, some controlled studies showed evidence of benefit in panic disorder (moclobemide is not available in some countries).

The use of benzodiazepines remains the subject of debate, given the risks of drowsiness, tolerance, and dependence: but many still consider benzodiazepines to be a reasonable first-line treatment in some patients, given the breadth of data supporting their use. Although the irreversible MAOI phenelzine is only used as a third-line drug due to its unfavourable side effect and interaction profile, it is considered very effective by clinicians (phenelzine is not available in all countries). The MAOI tranylcypromine has not been investigated in panic disorder.

When these treatment modalities have failed, drugs which have not been approved for panic disorder but which have showed promising results in preliminary studies can potentially be tried.

Some psychiatrists prefer switching before trying augmentation strategies, as when an additional drug is added to an ongoing treatment it is later sometimes difficult to determine which of the two drug regimens was the successful one. Moreover, combination therapy may be associated with increased side effects and interactions. Switching strategies, however, have the disadvantage that in some cases the first drug must be tapered off and the second must be introduced gradually because of possible adverse drug interactions, which may further delay remission.

3.12 **Psychological treatments in treatment-resistant cases**

Psychological treatments such as cognitive behaviour therapy (CBT) have to be considered in all patients, regardless of whether they are drug treatment non-responders or not. In studies without a control condition, patients having residual symptoms despite being on an adequate dose of medication showed improvement after the introduction of CBT (Heldt et al, 2003; Pollack et al, 1994). Conversely, SSRIs or clomipramine can improve patients who responded insufficiently to CBT, according to placebo-controlled studies (Hoffart et al, 1993; Kampman et al, 2002).

Adherence with drug treatment can be improved when the advantages and disadvantages of the drug are explained carefully to the patient, such as the delayed onset of effect or side effects like initial jitteriness. Patients with panic disorder sometimes express groundless or exaggerated fear of side effects of psychotropic drugs, such as addiction (even with drugs without known addiction potential).

Although efficacy of aerobic exercise was only moderate, it may be a useful adjunction to CBT and pharmacotherapy.

3.13 **Treating comorbid panic disorder**

If coexisting psychiatric disorders occur in patients with panic disorder, an effective treatment or combination of treatments that simultaneously addresses all disorders present should ideally be chosen. Untreated comorbid disorders can contribute to treatment failure if the chosen treatment does not have a broad spectrum of therapeutic activity. Unfortunately, not much data are available to guide treatment of comorbid panic disorder and other psychiatric disorders in this large group of patients, in part because agents are individually developed to treat specific disorders. Thus, the ideal strategies for treating panic disorder coexisting with other psychiatric disorders are currently speculative. The main strategy for pharmacological treatment is to choose an agent with effectiveness for both panic disorder and the additional conditions. Antidepressants have proven useful in this regard, because most conditions that occur in conjunction with panic disorder (e.g. major depression, social phobia and generalized anxiety disorder) appear to be responsive to these agents. Monotherapy with benzodiazepines would not be regarded as useful in patients with additional depression.

According to clinical experience, comorbid alcohol or substance abuse is much more difficult to treat than the panic part of the comorbid disorder. Even after panic symptomatology has been treated successfully, the addiction problem may still be there.

3.14 **Special populations**

The risks of drug treatment during pregnancy must be weighed against the risk of withholding treatment for panic disorder. Psychological interventions are probably preferable to pharmacological treatments in pregnant women. According to the majority of studies, the use of SSRIs and TCAs in pregnancy imposes no increased risk for malformations, although some reports have raised concerns about fetal cardiac effects, newborn persistent pulmonary hypertension, respiratory distress, and other effects. However, this is an emerging field and it pays to consult up-to-date information sources when making treatment decisions with pregnant women.

It is generally recommended to avoid paroxetine use among pregnant women or women planning to become pregnant if possible (ACOG, 2006). Pre-school-age children exposed to fluoxetine *in utero* did not show significant neurobehavioural changes (Goldstein and Sundell, 1999). The findings of a prospective controlled study suggest that long-term prenatal exposure to TCAs or fluoxetine does not adversely affect cognition, language development, or temperament (Nulman et al, 2002). The anticonvulsants valproate and carbamazepine, but not lamotrigine, were associated with an increased rate of congenital anomalies, as well as neonatal problems (Austin and Mitchell, 1998). An association between the use of benzodiazepines and congenital malformations has been reported (Laegreid et al, 1990). However, there has been no consistent proof that benzodiazepines may be hazardous. The available literature suggests that it is safe to take diazepam or chlordiazepoxide during pregnancy. It has been suggested that it would be prudent to avoid alprazolam during pregnancy (Iqbal et al, 2002). To avoid the potential risk of congenital defects, physicians should preferentially use those benzodiazepines that have the best safety records.

3.15 Breast feeding

SSRIs and TCAs are excreted into breast milk and low concentrations have been found in infants' serum (Simpson and Noble, 2000). A systematic review indicates that plasma levels of the SSRIs paroxetine and sertraline and the TCA nortriptyline in breast-fed infants levels are usually undetectable, whereas citalopram and fluoxetine produce infant plasma levels that are above 10% of the maternal plasma level in 22% and 17% of infants, respectively (Weissman et al, 2004). In mothers receiving TCAs (with the exception of doxepin), it seems unwarranted to recommend that breast feeding should be discontinued. Fluoxetine was associated with behaviour changes in two breast-fed infants. Treatment with other SSRIs (citalopram, fluvoxamine, paroxetine, or sertraline) seems to be compatible with breast feeding, although this view should be considered as preliminary due to the lack of data. Again it is important to consult up-to-date information sources when making treatment decisions with breast-feeding women.

Regarding anxiolytic benzodiazepines, adverse drug reactions in newborn infants have been described during maternal treatment with diazepam. During maternal treatment with all benzodiazepines, infants should be observed for signs of sedation, lethargy, poor suckling, and weight loss, and if high doses have to be used and long term administration is required, breast feeding should probably be discontinued (Iqbal et al, 2002; Spigset and Hägg, 1998).

3.16 Treating children and adolescents

The median onset of panic disorder is 24 years. Therefore, panic disorder in children and adolescents is relatively rare. Very limited data are available on pharmacological treatment of juvenile panic, and no randomized, controlled studies are available to date. For other anxiety disorders, a number of RCTs exists showing the efficacy of SSRIs and SNRIs in children and adolescents.

The potential benefits and risks of using SSRIs in children and adolescents with depression has been much debated, and there have been warnings against their use due to concerns about increased risk of suicidal ideation and behaviour (Hetrick et al, 2007; Scahill et al, 2005). However, some analyses found that SSRIs exhibit efficacy for treatment of depression in children and adolescents (Sharp and Hellings, 2006) and found no significant increase in risk of suicide or serious suicide attempt after starting treatment with newer antidepressant drugs (Simon et al, 2006). Concerns regarding major depression may not necessarily apply to the treatment of children and adolescents with anxiety disorders, because the risk of self-harm is less and the balance of therapeutic benefits and risks may differ. Nevertheless, careful monitoring is advisable, due to possible diagnostic uncertainty and the presence of comorbid depression. Some clinicians also think that it may be preferable to reserve pharmacological treatments for patients who do not respond to evidence-based psychological approaches.

3.17 Treatment of the elderly

The symptoms of panic disorder tend to decrease after the age of approximately 45 years. Therefore, panic disorder is relatively rare in elderly patients. However, panic attacks may occur in elderly patients with major depression. Few studies exist that investigate the treatment of anxiety disorders in the elderly. Escitalopram and citalopram appeared effective in reducing panic attack frequency in a small sample of elderly patients with recurrent panic attacks associated with a range of anxiety disorders (Rampello et al, 2006).

Factors that should be regarded in the treatment of the elderly include an increased sensitivity for anticholinergic properties of drugs, an increased risk for orthostatic hypotension and ECG changes, impaired memory, and possible paradoxical reactions to benzodiazepines (Lader and Morton, 1991); these may include depression, with or without suicidal tendencies, phobias, aggressiveness, violent behaviour, and symptoms misdiagnosed as psychosis. Thus, treatment with TCAs or benzodiazepines is less favourable, while SSRIs, SNRIs, and moclobemide appear to be safe.

3.18 **Treatment of patients with cardiovascular disease**

TCAs are best avoided in patients with cardiac disease, as they can increase heart rate and QT interval, induce orthostatic hypotension, slow cardiac conduction, and have significant quinidine-like effects on conduction within the myocardium. By contrast, the SSRIs have minimal effects on cardiovascular function and may have potentially beneficial effects on platelet aggregation (Davies et al, 2004; Roose, 2003). Potential cardiovascular side effects from venlafaxine must be considered. In a study with depressed patients aged 60 and older, venlafaxine was well tolerated. However, undesirable cardiovascular effects occurred in some of the participants (Johnson et al, 2006). Another study of depressed patients on high dose venlafaxine (mean 346 mg; range 225–525 mg) did not demonstrate any clinical or statistically significant effects on electrocardiographic (ECG) parameters (Mbaya et al, 2007).

3.19 **Novel treatment approaches**

Although many drugs are available for the treatment of panic disorder, the overall response rates leave much room for improvement, and the differences between active drugs and placebo are still only moderate. In order to improve treatment for anxiety disorders, many novel treatment approaches are currently under investigation. Unmet needs are antipanic drugs that have a faster onset than currently available antidepressants, higher response rates, no addiction potential, and less side effects. Putative future anxiolytic drugs currently under development are listed in Box 3.2.

Box 3.2 Putative future anxiolytics
Neurokinin receptor antagonists
Metabotropic glutamate (mGlu) type 2 receptor agonists
Serotonin receptor agonists and antagonists
Sigma ligands
Neuropeptide Y/S agonists
adenosine A_1 and A_2 receptor agonists
CRH receptor antagonists
Natriuretic peptide
Nitroflavonoids

References and further reading

ACOG (2006). ACOG Committee Opinion No. 354: Treatment with selective serotonin reuptake inhibitors during pregnancy. *Obstet Gynecol* **108**: 1601–3.

Austin MPV, Mitchell PB (1998). Psychotropic medications in pregnant women: treatment dilemmas. *Medical Journal of Australia* **169**: 428–431.

Bandelow B (1999). *Panic and Agoraphobia Scale (PAS)*. Hogrefe & Huber Publishers, Göttingen/Bern/Toronto/Seattle

Bandelow B, Stein DJ, Dolberg OT, Andersen HF, Baldwin DS (2007). Improvement of quality of life in panic disorder with escitalopram, citalopram, or placebo. *Pharmacopsychiatry* **40**: 152–6.

Bandelow B, Zohar J, Hollander E, et al. (2008). World Federation of Societies of Biological Psychiatry (WFSBP) guidelines for the pharmacological treatment of anxiety, obsessive-compulsive and post-traumatic stress disorders - first revision. *World J Biol Psychiatry* **9**: 248–312.

Davies SJ, Jackson PR, Potokar J, Nutt DJ (2004). Treatment of anxiety and depressive disorders in patients with cardiovascular disease. *Bmj* **328**: 939–43.

Goldstein DJ, Sundell K (1999). A review of the safety of selective serotonin reuptake inhibitors during pregnancy. *Human Psychopharmacology-Clinical and Experimental* **14**: 319–324.

Heldt E, Manfro GG, Kipper L, et al. (2003). Treating medication-resistant panic disorder: predictors and outcome of cognitive-behavior therapy in a Brazilian public hospital. *Psychother Psychosom* **72**: 43–8.

Hetrick S, Merry S, McKenzie J, Sindahl P, Proctor M (2007). Selective serotonin reuptake inhibitors (SSRIs) for depressive disorders in children and adolescents. *Cochrane Database Syst Rev* CD004851.

Hoffart A, Due-Madsen J, Lande B, Gude T, Bille H, Torgersen S (1993). Clomipramine in the treatment of agoraphobic inpatients resistant to behavioral therapy. *J Clin Psychiatry* **54**: 481–7.

Iqbal MM, Sobhan T, Ryals T (2002). Effects of commonly used benzodiazepines on the fetus, the neonate, and the nursing infant. *Psychiatr Serv* **53**: 39–49.

Johnson EM, Whyte E, Mulsant BH, Pollock BG, Weber E, Begley AE, Reynolds CF (2006). Cardiovascular changes associated with venlafaxine in the treatment of late-life depression. *Am J Geriatr Psychiatry* **14**: 796–802.

Kampman M, Keijsers GP, Hoogduin CA, Hendriks GJ (2002). A randomized, double-blind, placebo-controlled study of the effects of adjunctive paroxetine in panic disorder patients unsuccessfully treated with cognitive-behavioral therapy alone. *J Clin Psychiatry* **63**: 772–7.

Lader M, Morton S (1991). Benzodiazepine problems. *Br J Addict* **86**: 823–8.

Laegreid L, Olegard R, Conradi N, Hagberg G, Wahlstrom J, Abrahamsson L (1990). Congenital malformations and maternal consumption of benzodiazepines: a case-control study. *Dev Med Child Neurol* **32**: 432–41.

Mbaya P, Alam F, Ashim S, Bennett D (2007). Cardiovascular effects of high dose venlafaxine XL in patients with major depressive disorder. *Hum Psychopharmacol* **22**: 129–33.

Michelson D, Allgulander C, Dantendorfer K, et al. (2001). Efficacy of usual antidepressant dosing regimens of fluoxetine in panic disorder: randomised, placebo-controlled trial. *Br J Psychiatry* **179**: 514–8.

Nulman I, Rovet J, Stewart DE, Wolpin J, Pace-Asciak P, Shuhaiber S, Koren G (2002). Child development following exposure to tricyclic antidepressants or fluoxetine throughout fetal life: a prospective, controlled study. *Am J Psychiatry* **159**: 1889–95.

Pollack MH, Otto MW, Kaspi SP, Hammerness PG, Rosenbaum JF (1994). Cognitive behavior therapy for treatment-refractory panic disorder. *J Clin Psychiatry* **55**: 200–5.

Rampello L, Alvano A, Raffaele R, Malaguarnera M, Vecchio I (2006). New possibilities of treatment for panic attacks in elderly patients: escitalopram versus citalopram. *J Clin Psychopharmacol* **26**: 67–70.

Roose SP (2003). Treatment of depression in patients with heart disease. *Biol Psychiatry* **54**: 262–8.

Scahill L, Hamrin V, Pachler ME (2005). The use of selective serotonin reuptake inhibitors in children and adolescents with major depression. *J Child Adolesc Psychiatr Nurs* **18**: 86–9.

Seedat S, van Rheede van Oudtshoorn E, Muller JE, Mohr N, Stein DJ (2003). Reboxetine and citalopram in panic disorder: a single-blind, cross-over, flexible-dose pilot study. *Int Clin Psychopharmacol* **18**: 279–84.

Sharp SC, Hellings JA (2006). Efficacy and safety of selective serotonin reuptake inhibitors in the treatment of depression in children and adolescents: practitioner review. *Clin Drug Investig* **26**: 247–55.

Simon GE, Savarino J, Operskalski B, Wang PS (2006). Suicide risk during antidepressant treatment. *Am J Psychiatry* **163**: 41–7.

Simpson K, Noble S (2000). Fluoxetine - A review of its use in women's health. *Cns Drugs* **14**: 301–328.

Spigset O, Hägg S (1998). Excretion of psychotropic drugs into breast milk - Pharmacokinetic overview and therapeutic implications. *Cns Drugs* **9**: 111–134.

Weissman AM, Levy BT, Hartz AJ, Bentler S, Donohue M, Ellingrod VL, Wisner KL (2004). Pooled analysis of antidepressant levels in lactating mothers, breast milk, and nursing infants. *Am J Psychiatry* **161**: 1066–78.

Chapter 4

Non-pharmacological treatment

Key points

- Cognitive behaviour therapy is effective for panic disorder and agoraphobia
- Exposure therapy is a key component for patients with agoraphobia
- While drug treatment and CBT showed similar efficacy, a combination of psychopharmacological and psychological treatment is probably more effective than either monotherapy

---

4.1 Introduction

All patients with panic disorder require supportive interviews and attention to emotional states. Although there is no definition of 'counselling' techniques, as there are no manuals and no controlled treatment studies, many psychiatrists or general practitioners intuitively apply some kind of counselling in patients with panic attacks. Psychoeducative methods, including information about the nature and aetiology of panic disorder and agoraphobia, and the mechanism of action of psychological and drug treatments are a part of this treatment programme, as well as correcting misbeliefs about the origin of panic symptoms, and encouraging patients not to avoid feared situations.

Without being a professional psychotherapist, many physicians in primary care take advantage of the non-specific psychotherapy effects, by listening to the patient in a friendly, empathetic, and understanding conversation.

However, many patients may require specific psychological treatment interventions. Due to the high placebo effect in panic disorder, only psychological treatments that have been examined in randomized controlled trials (RCTs) should be used. Demonstration of efficacy should not only be based on a waiting list control, but also on comparisons with a 'psychological placebo' in order to show that treatment effects go significantly beyond the non-specific treatment effects that may emerge in friendly, empathetic, and understanding conversation of a physician or psychologist.

4.2 Psychoeducation

Even without specific psychotherapeutic interventions, 'psychoeducation' can be used in primary care. It includes information about the aetiology and treatment of panic attacks. The nature of panic disorder and agoraphobia should be explained to the patient:

1. Panic attacks are an inadequate 'fight or flight reaction' occurring without a natural threat
2. All symptoms can be explained by normal reactions to a dangerous situation, and do not mean a malfunction of body systems
3. Panic attacks are self-limiting
4. Panic symptoms such as increased heartbeat cannot lead to death or health damage, as all symptoms are natural reactions. For example, blood pressure and heart rate are only slightly increased or within the upper normal range
5. In the case of a panic attack, immediate help by a physician is not required
6. It is unnecessary to avoid situations in which medical help may not be available in the event of having an unexpected or situationally predisposed panic attack
7. Feared situations should not be avoided; avoidance will increase the fear of these situations.

4.3 Cognitive behaviour therapy

The most common non-pharmacological therapy used in the management of panic disorder is cognitive behaviour therapy (CBT). CBT was investigated in several controlled studies. In the majority of studies, cognitive-behavioural techniques were superior to waiting list control condition, to a pill placebo or a psychological placebo in panic disorder and/or agoraphobia (Bandelow et al, 2008).

CBT is an exposure-based approach aimed at helping patients reacquire a sense of safety around cues associated with panic disorder. CBT has two components: identifying and changing the distorted thinking patterns that maintain anxiety (cognitive therapy), and desensitizing anxiety through exposure to feared situations (behaviour therapy).

According to cognitive theories, panic symptoms are a consequence of cognitive distortions and an enduring tendency to misinterpret benign bodily sensations as indications of an immediately impending physical catastrophe. CBT is designed to help the patient understand the role of his or her cognitions in the development of panic and to accept a more benign interpretation of the bodily sensations.

The cognitive procedures include:

• Educating the patient about the symptoms of anxiety
• Identifying cognitive distortions, illogical ideas, and negative perceptions
• Cognitive restructuring to help patients disconfirm their negative predictions about the consequences of their symptoms.

Examples of the re-interpretation of cognitive biases are given in Table 4.1.

Agoraphobic avoidance is treated with progressive exposure to panic attack triggers. Starting with the most anxiety provoking situation, fear stimuli are put in a hierarchy, and efforts are made to tackle those feared situations which are least disabling, before

Table 4.1 Cognitive behaviour therapy: examples for re-interpretation of cognitive biases	
Patient's catastrophic misinterpretation	Alternative positive interpretation
Rapid heartbeat means that I might have a heart attack or heart failure	Rapid heartbeat is a normal symptom of physiological arousal, mobilizing the body for fight or flight
Tightness in the chest or throat or rapid breathing may lead to choking	In a fight or flight reaction, hyperventilation is a normal reaction in order to increase oxygen content in the blood
Light-headedness is a sign for being on the verge of fainting	Fainting is caused by a sudden drop in blood pressure, whereas in panic attacks, the blood pressure goes slightly up, making fainting an impossibility
I might lose control and do something rash or impulsive, such as losing control of the car, or jumping from a balcony	People experiencing a panic attack are in a state of high attention and are actually more in control than they need to be
Although I have experienced many panic attacks before without having any negative consequences, during the next panic attack something really serious could happen	All panic attacks have more or less a uniform symptomatology, and cannot lead to bodily harm

moving up the hierarchy. Exposure guided by therapists is more effective than a pro-gramme in which exposure is simply instructed (Gloster et al, 2011).

As many panic attacks occur 'out of the blue', they cannot be addressed by direct exposure therapy. Cognitive strategies have been developed to address spontaneous panic attacks. These include strategies for habituating the patient to panic symptoms. For instance in a breathing exercise, hyperventilation is provoked by some therapists; or, by turning the patient around quickly on the office chair of the psychotherapist, dizziness is induced.

CBT treatment sessions are highly structured. An agenda is agreed at the start of each session, and repeated belief ratings are used to monitor within-session cognitive change. In addition, frequent summaries are used to guarantee mutual understanding. At the end of each session a series of homework assignments are agreed upon as well.

Most controlled studies with CBT in panic disorder employed weekly sessions over 12–15 weeks. However, in daily clinical practice, patients often have 25–50 sessions, or more.

Although usually the gains are sustained maintained after ending the therapy ses-sions, relapses may occur and some patients will need 'booster sessions' to refresh therapeutic gains.

4.4 **Psychodynamic (psychoanalytic) therapy**

There only few studies employing psychodynamic psychotherapy in panic disorder. In one study, the authors reported psychodynamic therapy to be superior to 'applied relaxation' (Milrod et al, 2007), but the study is inconclusive due to problematic dealing with missing values due to attrition. Moreover, applied relaxation is a therapist-aided relaxation technique, which does not involve systematic therapeutic conversation. In another study with many methodological problems, pure psychodynamic therapy was less effective than a combination of psychodynamic therapy and exposure in agoraphobic patients (Hoffart and Martinsen, 1990). In one study psychodynamic treatment was significantly less effective than CBT (Beutel et al, 2012). Before psychodynamic therapy can be recommended for routine treatment, further studies are needed.

4.5 Other treatments

Two methodologically problematic studies assessed the efficacy of client-centred therapy. In the first study (Teusch et al, 1997), patients with panic disorder and agoraphobia were assigned to pure client-centred therapy (CCT) or to additional behavioural exposure treatment. For a short period, the combined treatment was superior in patients' coping actively with anxiety and improving agoraphobic symptoms. The second study did not find a difference between both groups (Teusch et al, 2001). As the studies did not involve a control group and did not have enough power to detect treatment differences, their scientific validity is limited.

Relaxation techniques are often proposed to patients with panic disorder. However, there is not enough evidence from adequately controlled trials to support any relaxation technique.

In progressive muscle relaxation, the client is taught to relax progressively by alternately tensing and relaxing muscles while lying in a comfortable position. The method seems to be less effective than CBT (Marks et al, 1983). Results with autogenic training in patients with anxiety disorders were mixed (Jorm et al, 2004), and methodologically sound RCTs are lacking. Biofeedback and hypnosis were not investigated in panic disorder.

Other psychological treatments have not been found superior to control interventions, or have not been subject to controlled investigations.

4.6 Side effects of psychotherapy

Although psychological treatments do not lead to side effects in the generally understood sense, certain negative effects may be associated with psychotherapy:

- According to studies, up to 25% of patients with panic disorder refuse to participate in exposure programmes
- As with pharmacological approaches, it should be emphasized that response is not immediate
- Prolonged courses are often needed to maintain an initial treatment response
- Dependence on the therapist may occur, with problems when treatment is stopped.

4.7 Exercise

Exercise has been proposed as a remedy for all kinds of psychiatric disorders; however, only few controlled studies have been performed to assess its usefulness. In the first study examining the role of exercise in an anxiety disorder, patients with panic disorder were randomly assigned to three treatment modalities: running, clomipramine, or placebo. Both exercise and clomipramine led to a significant decrease of symptoms in comparison to placebo; however, exercise was still significantly less effective than clomipramine (Bandelow et al, 2000). In a subsequent study, a combination of drug treatment and exercise was investigated. Patients received paroxetine or placebo in a double-blind manner. Additionally, patients from both groups were randomly allocated to exercise and a control group, relaxation training. Whereas paroxetine was superior to placebo, exercise did not differ from the control group, perhaps due to the high effect sizes obtained in the latter treatment modality. Taking the results of both studies together, exercise seems to have some effect in panic disorder; however, this effect seems to be less pronounced than the effect of medication (Wedekind et al, 2007).

4.8 **Repetitive transcranial magnetic stimulation**

Repetitive transcranial magnetic stimulation (rTMS) is a non-invasive modality that raised some hopes in the treatment of major depression. However, it could not consistently be shown that the method was superior to sham application as a control group. Likewise, in panic disorder, low frequency rTMS administered over the right dorsolateral prefrontal cortex did not differ from sham rTMS as an add-on to serotonin reuptake inhibitors (Prasko et al, 2006).

4.9 **Combination of psychotherapy and drug treatment**

Psychological and pharmacological treatment modalities must be seen as partners, not alternatives, in the treatment of panic disorder.

There is conflicting evidence regarding the comparative efficacy of both modalities and the role of combination therapies. In order to avoid possible biases due to different study conditions, we conducted a meta-analysis of only those studies that included both a pharmacological treatment, a psychological treatment, or combinations of both within one study design, so that patients were randomly assigned to different treatment conditions realized within each study (Bandelow et al, 2007). In this meta-analysis, it was shown that the effect sizes for psychological and pharmacological approaches were similar in the acute treatment of panic disorder and a combination of both modalities was more effective that CBT or drug treatment alone (Bandelow et al, 2007). Moreover, when looking at direct comparisons of both modalities, the majority of studies supported the superiority of combination therapy over both modalities (Bandelow et al, 2008).

When deciding whether drug treatment, psychotherapy, or a combination of both should be recommended, other considerations have to be taken into account. It is generally assumed that after treatment termination, CBT is associated with sustained effects, while relapses occur soon after stopping drug treatment. However, most follow-up studies do not find significant differences in relapse rates between CBT and drugs (Bandelow et al, 2008). With drug treatment, adverse events can occur, but also CBT is not accepted by all patients, because it is time consuming and may be associated with distress caused by exposure strategies. According to a meta-analysis, drop-out rates are the same in pharmacological and psychological treatment studies (Mitte, 2005). CBT is more expensive than drug treatment and is not readily available in many parts of the world. Even in centres with a high accessibility to behaviour therapists, it may take several months to obtain a place on the treatment list, a period in which improvement usually occurs with drug therapy. In the case that treatment with one drug fails, there are several alternative drug treatment options, increasing the chance for remission for an individual patient, whereas after a failure of CBT other psychological treatment options are lacking.

For these reasons, patients should be offered a choice of treatment approaches, selection being affected by patient clinical features, needs and preference, and by the local availability of services able to offer evidence-based psychological interventions.

Pharmacotherapy and psychotherapy may work synergistically. It remains speculative as to where psychotherapy exerts its action in the brain. However, it seems unlikely that psychotherapy can directly influence the relatively primitive, innate anxiety programmes that are driven by the thalamus and the amygdala, as these are present in all mammals. It is probable that psychological treatment strategies address higher cognitive centres. For example, the fears of panic patients involve general knowledge about medical conditions (such as: 'a myocardial infarction is characterized by symptoms such as fast or irregular heart beat, chest pain, or dyspnoea'). These considerations require brain centres with higher cognitive abilities. These centres are probably located in the prefrontal cortex. In panic anxiety, these 'intelligent' centres are overridden by primitive fear mechanisms. By strengthening the ability of the higher centres to control archaic fear mechanisms, cognitive therapy may reduce anxiety. Antidepressants, on the other hand, increase firing of serotonergic neurons projecting from the raphe nuclei to the primitive anxiety network structures such as the amygdala, thalamus, locus coeruleus, and others (but they also influence the prefrontal cortex). Therefore it may be assumed that psychotherapy and drugs work synergistically by exerting their action in different brain centres.

4.10 **Self-help**

Patient preference and the suboptimal effects of pharmacological or psychological treatment approaches have encouraged the development of a range of self-help techniques and therapies in anxiety disorders. However, there have been relatively few randomized controlled trials of the efficacy and acceptability of self-help approaches and few studies have been conducted in diagnostically homogenous groups, with reliable outcome measures and robust statistical analysis. These methods included self-help by reading books (bibliotherapy) (Lidren et al, 1994) and computer-guided CBT therapy (Carlbring et al, 2006). However, the UK National Institute for Health and Care Excellence concluded that there was insufficient evidence to recommend the general introduction of computerized cognitive behaviour therapy for anxiety symptoms or disorders (NICE, 2007).

Many self-help groups exist for patients with anxiety disorders. In these groups patients may find emotional support by other sufferers and may exchange experiences about helpful treatments and specialist centres.

4.11 Sick notes and disability pension

Many patients with panic disorder have a tendency to go on sick leave, as they have the feeling that they need to take it easy. However, usually panic symptomatology does not get better when a patient is on sick leave, and agoraphobia may even get worse when the patient is not confronted with his normal surroundings.

Also, some patients insist on going into early retirement in the hope of finding relief from their symptoms. However, according to clinical experience, panic attacks and avoidance of feared situations do not improve in these cases, but may even take a chronic course in early pensioners. Very frequently, patients are pensioned at a relatively early age due to panic disorder, but not all options for treatment-refractory cases have yet been exhausted. Sometimes even standard treatments like CBT or selective serotonin reuptake inhibitors have never been used. Therefore, early retirement may only be indicated in few patients, such as those with comorbid disorders.

References and further reading

Bandelow B (1999). *Panic and Agoraphobia Scale (PAS)*. Hogrefe & Huber Publishers, Göttingen/Bern/Toronto/Seattle

Bandelow B, Broocks A, Pekrun G, et al. (2000). The use of the Panic and Agoraphobia Scale (P & A) in a controlled clinical trial. *Pharmacopsychiatry* **33**: 174–81.

Bandelow B, Seidler-Brandler U, Becker A, Wedekind D, Rüther E (2007). Meta-analysis of randomized controlled comparisons of psychopharmacological and psychological treatments for anxiety disorders. *World J Biol Psychiatry* **8**: 175–87.

Bandelow B, Zohar J, Hollander E, et al. (2008). World Federation of Societies of Biological Psychiatry (WFSBP) guidelines for the pharmacological treatment of anxiety, obsessive-compulsive and post-traumatic stress disorders - first revision. *World J Biol Psychiatry* **9**: 248–312.

Beutel ME, Stark R, Pan H, Silbersweig DA, Dietrich S (2012). Langzeitergebnisse einer Funktionellen-Magnetresonanztomographie-Studie. *Psychotherapeut* **57**: 227–233.

Carlbring P, Bohman S, Brunt S, Buhrman M, Westling BE, Ekselius L, Andersson G (2006). Remote treatment of panic disorder: a randomized trial of internet-based cognitive behavior therapy supplemented with telephone calls. *Am J Psychiatry* **163**: 2119–25.

Gloster AT, Wittchen HU, Einsle F, et al. (2011). Psychological treatment for panic disorder with agoraphobia: A randomized controlled trial to examine the role of therapist-guided exposure in situ in CBT. *J Consult Clin Psychol* **79**: 406–20.

Hoffart A, Martinsen EW (1990). Exposure-based integrated vs pure psychodynamic treatment of agoraphobic inpatients. *Psychotherapy* **27**: 210–218.

Jorm AF, Christensen H, Griffiths KM, Parslow RA, Rodgers B, Blewitt KA (2004). Effectiveness of complementary and self-help treatments for anxiety disorders. *Med J Aust* **181**: S29–46.

Lidren DM, Watkins PL, Gould RA, Clum GA, Asterino M, Tulloch HL (1994). A comparison of bibliotherapy and group therapy in the treatment of panic disorder. *J Consult Clin Psychol* **62**: 865–9.

Marks IM, Gray S, Cohen D, Hill R, Mawson D, Ramm E, Stern RS (1983). Imipramine and brief therapists-aided exposure in agoraphobics having self-exposure homework. *Arch Gen Psychiatry* **40**: 153–62.

Milrod B, Leon AC, Busch F, et al. (2007). A randomized controlled clinical trial of psychoanalytic psychotherapy for panic disorder. *Am J Psychiatry* **164**: 265–72.

Mitte K (2005). A meta-analysis of the efficacy of psycho- and pharmacotherapy in panic disorder with and without agoraphobia. *J Affect Disord* **88**: 27–45.

National Institute for Health and Clinical Excellence (NICE) (2007). Anxiety (amended): Management of Anxiety (Panic Disorder, with or without Agoraphobia, and Generalised Anxiety Disorder) in Adults in Primary, Secondary and Community Care. NICE, London.

Prasko J, Paskova B, Zalesky R, Novak T, Kopecek M, Bares M, Horacek J (2006). The effect of repetitive transcranial magnetic stimulation (rTMS) on symptoms in obsessive compulsive disorder. A randomized, double blind, sham controlled study. *Neuro Endocrinol Lett* **27**: 327–32.

Teusch L, Bohme H, Gastpar M (1997). The benefit of an insight-oriented and experiential approach on panic and agoraphobia symptoms. Results of a controlled comparison of client-centered therapy alone and in combination with behavioral exposure. *Psychother Psychosom* **66**: 293–301.

Teusch L, Bohme H, Finke J (2001). [Conflict-centered individual therapy or integration of psychotherapy methods. Process of change in client-centered psychotherapy with and without behavioral exposure therapy in agoraphobia with panic disorder]. *Nervenarzt* **72**: 31–9.

Wedekind D, Broocks A, Weiss N, Rotter-Glattkowski P, Engel K, Neubert K, Bandelow B (2007). Controlled study for effectiveness of sport vs. relaxation training in combination with paroxetine vs. Placebo in the treatment of the panic disorder. *Nervenarzt* **78**: 510–10.

Conclusions

Panic disorder is a common and disabling disorder. In most cases drug treatment and cognitive behaviour therapy may substantially improve quality of life. Due to increased efforts in the systematic clinical evaluation of psychopharmacological agents in the treatment of anxiety in the recent years, a comprehensive database has been collected so that precise recommendations can be provided for treating panic disorder.

The drugs recommended as the first-line treatment for panic disorder are the selective serotonin reuptake inhibitors (SSRIs) or the serotonin norepinephrine reuptake inhibitor (SNRI) venlafaxine. Tricyclic antidepressants such as imipramine or clomipramine are also effective in panic disorder, but due to their more unfavourable side effect profile as compared with the SSRIs or SNRIs, these drugs are reserved for second or third-line treatment. In treatment-resistant cases, benzodiazepines like alprazolam may be used when the patient does not have a history of dependency and tolerance. Benzodiazepines can be combined with antidepressants in the first weeks of treatment before the onset of efficacy of the antidepressants. The irreversible monoamine oxidase inhibitor phenelzine is also effective in panic disorder, but its use should be restricted to otherwise treatment-resistant cases because of possible dangerous side effects and interactions. A number of treatment options exist for patients who are non-responsive to standard treatments.

Cognitive-behavioural therapy (CBT) has approximately the same effect size as drug therapy. The combination of CBT and drug therapy is more effective than both modalities alone.

Appendix 1

The history of the diagnosis of panic disorder

In Appendix Table 1.1, a short synopsis of the diagnosis of panic disorder is given. Although it is often assumed that panic disorder is a vogue of the 'modern times', it seems obvious that the disorder always existed and is relatively independent of cultural and epochal influences.

Table 1.1 History of the diagnosis of panic disorder	
600 BC	The Greek poet Sappho describes a panic attack in a poem.
1621	The English author and clergyman Robert Burton describes panic attacks in 'Anatomy of Melancholy'.
1850	The Japanese physician Gen'yu Imaizumi describes a patient with panic attacks (*hossasei shinkei-sho*) who was treated with 'confrontation', 'persuasion', and 'paradoxical interventions'.
1866	The French psychiatrist Morel describes the syndrome as *délire émotif*, a disturbance of the autonomic nervous system.
1871	The American military physician Da Costa describes the condition as due to an 'irritable heart'.
1872	The German psychiatrist Westphal coins the expression 'agoraphobia' for patients with panic attacks and fear of crowded places.
1892	The Russian physiologist Ivan Pavlov describes the phenomenon of classical conditioning, on which early learning theories are based.
1895	The Austrian neuropathologist Sigmund Freud coins the term 'anxiety neurosis', describes panic attacks and agoraphobia and develops psychoanalytic theories on the origin of pathological anxiety.
1920	The American psychologists John Broadus Watson and Rosalie Rayner develop models of human fear conditioning.
1938	The American psychologist Burrhus Frederic Skinner discovers operant conditioning, on which first behavioural treatment approaches are based.
1959	The American psychiatrist Donald F. Klein coins the term 'panic disorder' and conducts the first double-blind study with the tricyclic antidepressant imipramine
1966	The British psychiatrist Isaac Marks suggests exposure therapy for agoraphobia

(continued)

Table 1.1 History of the diagnosis of panic disorder	
1967	The American scientists Ferris Pitts and John McClure show increased sensitivity to lactate infusion in patients with panic disorder, thus first showing that neurobiological dysfunctions may underlie anxiety disorders.
1970	The American psychologist Aaron T. Beck develops cognitive behaviour treatment for panic disorder.
1978	The term 'panic disorder' is introduced in the 'Research Diagnostic Criteria', a predecessor of DSM-II.
2000	The American psychiatrist Jack Gorman describes the 'Anxiety Network', an integrative neurobiological model of pathological fear in humans.

Appendix 2

PANIC AND AGORAPHOBIA SCALE (PAS)
Clinician-Rated Version
B. Bandelow

Patient:

Rater: **Date:**   **Visit:**

Study Nr.

Rate the past week!

A) panic attacks
A.1. Frequency
- ❏ 0   no panic attack in the past week
- ❏ 1   1 panic attack in the past week
- ❏ 2   2 or 3 panic attacks in the past week
- ❏ 3   4 - 6 panic attacks in the past week
- ❏ 4   more than 6 panic attacks in the past week

A.2. Severity
- ❏ 0   no panic attacks
- ❏ 1   attacks were usually very mild
- ❏ 2   attacks were usually moderate
- ❏ 3   attacks were usually severe
- ❏ 4   attacks were usually extremely severe

A.3. Average duration of panic attacks
- ❏ 0   no panic attacks
- ❏ 1   1 to 10 minutes
- ❏ 2   over 10 to 60 minutes
- ❏ 3   over 1 to 2 hours
- ❏ 4   over 2 hours and more

U. Were most of the attacks expected (occurring in feared situations) or unexpected (spontaneous)?
- ❏ 9   no panic attacks

❏ 0 mostly unexpected	❏ 1 more unexpected than expected	❏ 2 some unexpected, some expected	❏ 3 more expected than unexpected	❏ 4 mostly expected

B) Agoraphobia, avoidance behaviour
B.1. Frequency of avoidance behaviour
- ❏ 0   no avoidance (or no agoraphobia)
- ❏ 1   infrequent avoidance of feared situations
- ❏ 2   occasional avoidance of feared situations
- ❏ 3   frequent avoidance of feared situations
- ❏ 4   very frequent avoidance of feared situations

B.2. Number of feared situations
How many situations are avoided or induce panic attacks or discomfort?
- ❏ 0   none (or no agoraphobia)
- ❏ 1   1 situation
- ❏ 2   2 - 3 situations
- ❏ 3   4 - 8 situations
- ❏ 4   occurred in very many different situations

B.3. Importance of avoided situations
How important are the avoided situations?
- ❏ 0   unimportant (or no agoraphobia)
- ❏ 1   not very important
- ❏ 2   moderately important
- ❏ 3   very important
- ❏ 4   extremely important

C) Anticipatory anxiety ("fear of fear")
C.1. Frequency of anticipatory anxiety
- ❏ 0   no fear of having a panic attack
- ❏ 1   infrequent fear of having a panic attack
- ❏ 2   sometimes fear of having a panic attack
- ❏ 3   frequent fear of having a panic attack
- ❏ 4   fear of having a panic attack all the time

C.2. How strong was this 'fear of fear'?
- ❏ 0   no
- ❏ 1   mild
- ❏ 2   moderate
- ❏ 3   marked
- ❏ 4   extreme

D) Disability
D.1. Disability in family relationships (partnership, children etc.)
- ❏ 0   no
- ❏ 1   mild
- ❏ 2   moderate
- ❏ 3   marked
- ❏ 4   extreme

D.2. Disability in social relationships and leisure time (social events like cinema etc.)
- ❏ 0   no
- ❏ 1   mild
- ❏ 2   moderate
- ❏ 3   marked
- ❏ 4   extreme

D.3. Disability in employment (or housework)
- ❏ 0   no
- ❏ 1   mild
- ❏ 2   moderate
- ❏ 3   marked
- ❏ 4   extreme

E) Worries about health
E.1. Worries about health damage
Patient was worried about suffering bodily damage due to the disorder
- ❏ 0   not true
- ❏ 1   hardly true
- ❏ 2   partly true
- ❏ 3   mostly true
- ❏ 4   definitely true

E.2. Assumption of organic disease
Patient thought that his anxiety symptoms are due to a somatic and not to a psychological disorder
- ❏ 0   not true, psychological disorder
- ❏ 1   hardly true
- ❏ 2   partly true
- ❏ 3   mostly true
- ❏ 4   definitely true, somatic disorder

Total score: Add all item scores except item U.

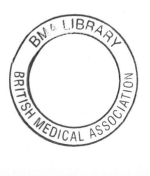

Index